THATCHER
versus
DOUGLAS

by

M.G Bucholtz, B.Sc., MBA, M.Sc.

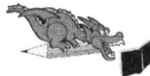

A Wood Dragon Book

THATCHER

versus

DOUGLAS

The CCF, the Liberals, and the
Mossbank Debate of 1957

by

M.G Bucholtz, B.Sc., MBA, M.Sc.

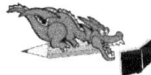

A Wood Dragon Book

Published by:
Wood Dragon Books
Box 429, Mossbank, Saskatchewan, Canada, S0H 3G0
http://www.wooddragonbooks.com

ISBN: 978-1-990863-34-9 (Paperback)
ISBN : 978-1-990863-41-7 (eBook)

To contact the author: supercyclereport@gmail.com

Acknowledgements

Many people assisted me in accessing vital research
material for this book. Special thanks to:

- Joan Bumphrey and Ken Kirkpatrick at the Mossbank
  Museum
- The research librarians at the Legislative Library of
  Saskatchewan
- Jeremy Patzer, MP for the Saskatchewan riding of
  Cypress Hills Grasslands, and his Ottawa staff
- Carla Beck, Leader of Saskatchewan's Opposition,
  MLA for Regina Lakeview, and her Regina staff.

Years in Office

T.C. DOUGLAS

Member of Parliament—Canada (CCF)
October 14, 1935—June 15, 1944
Weyburn

Member of the Legislative Assembly of Saskatchewan (CCF)
June 15, 1944—November 7, 1961
Weyburn

Premier of Saskatchewan (CCF)
June 15, 1944—November 7, 1961

Leader of The New Democratic Party—Canada (NDP)
August 3, 1961—April 24, 1971

Member of Parliament—Canada (NDP)
October 22, 1962—June 25, 1968
Burnaby-Coquitlam

Member of Parliament—Canada (NDP)
February 10, 1969—May 22, 1979
Nanaimo—Cowichan—The Islands

ROSS THATCHER

Member of Parliament—Canada (CCF)
June 11, 1945—August 10, 1953
Moose Jaw

Member of Parliament—Canada (CCF)
August 10, 1953—June 10, 1957
Moose Jaw—Lake Centre

Member of the Legislative Assembly of Saskatchewan (Liberal)
June 8, 1960—July 22, 1971
Morse

Premier of Saskatchewan (Liberal)
May 22, 1964—June 30, 1971

Contents

Introduction

I am not from Saskatchewan originally. I landed here in 1990 from Ontario. After graduating from Queen's University in 1986, my first job was in the Stelco steel mill in Hamilton, Ontario. But the smog and pollution belching from Hamilton's steel mills, was intolerable. I needed fresh air and open space. So, I bid adieu to Hamilton and set my sights on Regina and a position in the Research Centre at IPSCO.

In 1995, I met my future wife, a grain farmer's daughter, from south of Assiniboia, Saskatchewan. On our many visits to the Assiniboia area to see family, we would drive past the turnoff on Highway #2 leading into the town of Mossbank. Time and again, I would notice the wording on the road sign: *Home of the Great Debate.* Little did I know that one day these words would motivate me to write a book.

In 2020, we decided to leave Regina for a quieter lifestyle in the south country. After visiting numerous communities south of Moose Jaw, we decided to make Mossbank our new location. One day in early 2021, I had a phone call from an acquaintance in Regina. He asked where I had moved to. When I replied "Mossbank," there was a slight pause on the end of the line. Then he remarked, "Oh … Mossbank, the home of the Great Debate." My mind immediately flashed back to the road sign on Highway #2. I decided I needed to learn more about this historical event.

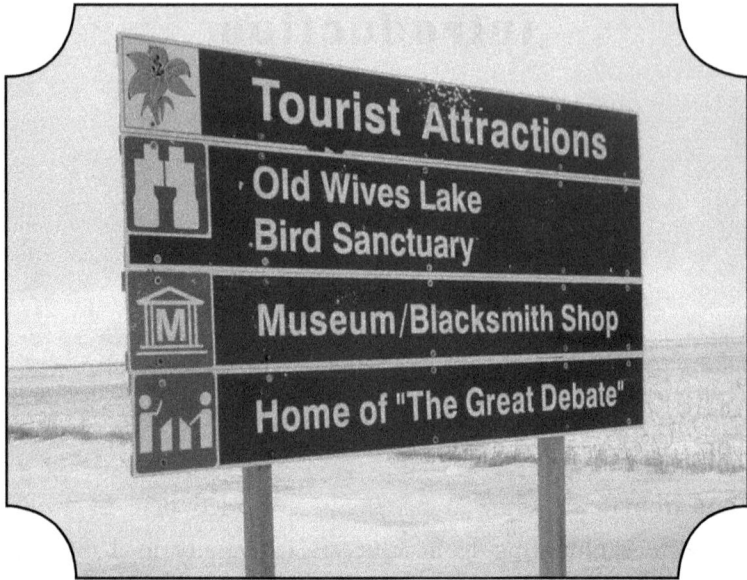

Highway sign advertising Mossbank as the Home of the Great Debate

As I searched the internet, I became fascinated with Tommy Douglas, Ross Thatcher and the fact that they had chosen the small village of Mossbank in 1957 to have their debate. Who were these politicians? Why 1957? Why Mossbank? My curiosity started to grow. Many of my questions, however, were not easily answered. I began to realize that the Great Debate was slowly being forgotten about.

In mid-2022, I approached Brian Howe, who happened to be the Mayor of Mossbank at the time, to discuss the 1957 Great Debate. He expressed enthusiasm for any efforts or events that might commemorate the event. I immediately began thinking about writing a book that would explore the political dynamic of 1950s Saskatchewan that culminated in the debate.

I combed through stacks of old papers at the Mossbank Museum with assistance from Joan Bumphrey and Ken Kirkpatrick. I reached out to area MP Jeremy Patzer who engaged his staff in Ottawa to locate historical facts and figures pertaining to Douglas, Thatcher, and the debate. My wife reached out to Carla Beck, Leader of Saskatchewan's Opposition, and MLA for Regina Lakeview, whose staff in Regina located a transcript copy of the debate.

This had been a debate about the Saskatchewan Crown Corporations, some of which had been launched by previous Liberal governments: Saskatchewan Power Corporation, Saskatchewan Telephones. The remaining Crown Corporations were started by the government of Premier Tommy Douglas following his ascension to the position of Premier in 1944: Saskatchewan Reconstruction Housing Corporation, Saskatchewan Fur Marketing Service, Saskatchewan Fish Marketing Board, Saskatchewan Government Airways, Saskatchewan Lake and Forest Corporation, Saskatchewan Box Factory, Saskatchewan Tannery Products, Saskatchewan Shoe Products, Saskatchewan Woollen Mill Products, Saskatchewan Minerals, Saskatchewan Horse Marketing Association, Saskatchewan Government Printing, Saskatchewan Radio Broadcasting, Saskatchewan Government Insurance, and Saskatchewan Transportation Corporation. I set out to learn about the circumstances that led the Douglas government to establish these Crowns. I set my sights on finding answers to the questions: who was Tommy Douglas? Who was Ross Thatcher? What life events shaped their political ideologies? How did the 1957 debate affect their political trajectories?

Researching this book was neither quick nor easy. I spent over 400 hours sifting through disparate bits of information gleaned from a wide diversity of sources, including a CBC documentary film, printed proceedings of legislative sittings from the 1940s and 1950s, and records of Saskatchewan and Canadian electoral results. I read political biographies and archival material to learn more about Thatcher, Douglas, and their respective political allies and opponents. I spent many days in the library at the

Saskatchewan Legislature gingerly thumbing my way through fragile, old Crown Corporation financial statements.

As I searched for information, I started to realize the task of researching the debate would be challenging. Those who codify history have a way of painting a one-dimensional perspective. Political figures can be made to look heroic; they can be also be given a villainous slant. With the passage of time, these perspectives can take on a permanency. In the case of Tommy Douglas, he has been cast as a giant of a man, and a great politician. As I delved into the backgrounds of Douglas and Thatcher, I ignored historical perspective. I aimed at arriving at my own opinion as to who they were and what had motivated them to meet for a debate in Mossbank in 1957.

My research was made more challenging when I realized that many of the information sources I had accessed had relegated the 1957 Debate to a mere footnote. Mossbank resident Ken Kirkpatrick was 14 years old at the time of the debate. One day, as I was sifting through old newspapers at the Mossbank Museum, he told me, "People came, they heard it, they saw it, and then they went home to get on with their lives."

Yet, the event is labelled as The Great Debate. The question that kept repeating in my mind was, why is it called the Great Debate? As I parsed the transcript of the debate, weighing Douglas's arguments, I started to piece it together, connecting the dots. This 1957 event was not just a debate. It *really* was a Great Debate. Prior to 1957, politics was generally conducted by individual candidates knocking on doors, giving speeches, and getting mentioned in whatever newspapers existed. The Great Debate marked a pivot point in politics. Two politicians came together in a public setting and exchanged viewpoints in a structured format with a moderator setting the tone. Reporters from far and wide were in attendance, broadcasting on radio and crafting written headline articles for newspapers. In Canada, political candidates exchanging viewpoints in front of the public and in front of media is the current paradigm. For the tipping point towards this paradigm, we need look no further than the Mossbank debate of 1957.

This book explores the family history of both Tommy Douglas and Ross Thatcher, the life events and experiences that shaped their political views, and their respective political experiences in Ottawa and in Regina. The history of the CCF Party and its founding principles as set down in the *Regina Manifesto* are explored (it would be these principles that led to the creation and structure of the Crown Corporations). The finances of these Crown entities are also explored in detail including the inference of there being two sets of accounting ledgers (that political opposition leaders in Saskatchewan often claim they will abolish when they become Premier – but never do). The political jockeying leading up to the debate then comes into focus. The entire transcript of the debate is presented, along with my critical analysis of the arguments expressed, to assist the reader in better understanding the issues that were raised during the debate.

Throughout the book, I take several off-ramps that lead the reader into deeper descriptions of the people and events that surrounded these two men, their careers, and their decisions. Following these off-ramps might led you to learning new things about Canadian politics, Saskatchewan politics, global geopolitical history, and even Saskatchewan Crown Corporations. The book concludes with an overview of the political paths taken by these two gentlemen in the years after the debate.

The Douglas years were a unique time in the political history of Saskatchewan; Mossbank on April 20, 1957 marked a key event in this history. Tommy Douglas and Ross Thatcher left an indelible impression on Saskatchewan. We may never see two politicians like them again.

May we never forget who they were, how they shaped this province, and how their showdown on May 20, 1957 changed politics as we knew it.

1

From Scotland,
Tommy Douglas Came

The story of Tommy Douglas begins in Falkirk, Scotland. The town of Falkirk is located 38 kilometers northwest of Edinburgh and 33 kilometers northeast of Glasgow, in the county of Stirlingshire. The name *Falkirk* has its linguistic origins in the Gaelic expression *Egglesbrech*, meaning speckled church. The original church in the settlement is said to have been made from a speckled variety of limestone. The Gaelic expression *Egglesbrech* eventually evolved into *Fawkirk* and then to the modern-day variation Falkirk.

The history of Scotland is a complex web of suspense, intrigue, conspiracy, religion, English royalty, and executioner's chopping blocks. This complex web intersects with Falkirk, Scotland which has lent its name to two significant battles: the First Battle of Falkirk and the Second Battle of Falkirk. These battles were not just isolated events. These battles were the culmination of complex political developments in Scottish history and speak to the desire of the Scottish people to stand up for themselves and to fight for what they thought was right. I cannot help but think that the fighting spirit woven into the fabric of Scottish history had a profound impact on the young Tommy Douglas. This fighting spirit would be on full display years later as he made a name for himself in Canadian politics.

THE FIRST BATTLE OF FALKIRK

The First Battle of Falkirk on July 22, 1298 was between the armies of William Wallace and Edward I of England. Relations between England and Scotland had been amicable for over 200 years, but any sense of friendliness came to an abrupt end when Edward I ascended to the throne of England. Edward's imposing height earned him the nickname Edward Longshanks. Also imposing, was his aggressive attitude toward expanding English rule. By 1283, he had conquered Wales and had brought it under his control. He then turned his sights on Scotland. Edward made it clear to the Scottish nobility that though they could govern themselves, he would have oversight and the final say in all matters. To ensure this oversight, he installed nobleman John de Balliol as King of Scotland after de Balliol pledged homage to Edward. Scottish nobility began applying pressure on de Balliol, urging him to align with Edward's enemy, King Philip IV of France, to help push back Edward and his authority over Scotland. John de Balliol's homage to Edward soon started to waver. Angered at this development, in 1296 Edward and his troops suddenly marched on Scotland – destroying the village of Berwick, sacking Edinburgh, and taking John de Balliol prisoner. Edward I then declared himself King of Scotland and Lord Superior of Scotland.

In the aftermath of this political upheaval, the Scottish people gave Edward the outward appearance of loyalty. Behind the scenes, it was a different story; the Scottish people were planning revenge. In 1297, military leader William Wallace staged a surprise attack on Edward's troops, pushing them back across the border into England. William Wallace was deemed a hero by the Scots and was named Guardian of Scotland.

In 1298, more determined than ever to crush Scottish resitance, Edward launched an offensive attack– the First Battle of Falkirk. Edward's offensive was successful; Wallace and his troops were soundly defeated and no longer would England and Scotland enjoy amicable relations. Wallace was removed from his Guardian position and imprisoned. Guardianship of Scotland was then bestowed jointly on nobleman Robert the Bruce and de Balliol's nephew, John Comyn. Even though Bruce had fought alongside William Wallace, he cleverly had managed to mend relations with Edward Longshanks.

In 1306, John Comyn was murdered and Robert the Bruce seized the throne, declaring himself the King of Scots. Edward I died of dysentery on the battlefield shortly afterward in 1307. His son, Edward II was never able to defeat Bruce's troops and Robert the Bruce remained on the Scottish throne until his death in 1329. Robert the Bruce was succeeded by his five-year-old son David II.

THE SECOND BATTLE

The next two hundred and fifty years were a back-and-forth drama of invasions, captures, mysterious deaths, executions, family squabbles, hostage takings, and shifting religious and political alliances. At the heart of all the intrigue was the House of Stewart (the name Stewart was eventually changed to Stuart).

In the mid-1500s, King James (Stuart) V of Scotland and his wife Madeline of France had a daughter, Mary. When she was merely six days old, her father was killed in battle and she was placed on the throne. Being too young to rule, Mary was sent to France to be properly educated. In her absence Madeline tended to the affairs of state with assistance from a variety of regents. Mary eventually returned to Scotland, assumed her place on the throne, and married her English cousin, Henry Stuart (Lord Darnley). The political drama then resumed in earnest. Mary gave birth to a son, James Stuart. Darnley was shortly thereafter killed in a mysterious explosion. It came to light that Mary had a lover, the Earl of Bothwell. Fingers were soon pointed at the Earl as a suspect in the explosion. Mary was accused of being an accomplice and was forced off the throne. Her son James (at the age of thirteen months) was placed on the throne. Mary and the Earl were imprisoned, but Mary escaped and fled to England where she sought refuge with her first cousin Queen Elizabeth I. Mayhem and controversy followed Mary to London where fingers soon pointed at her as the mastermind behind rumored plans to dethrone her cousin Elizabeth. Certainly, the untimely death of Elizabeth would have worked to Mary's advantage; Elizabeth was unmarried and had no successors waiting in line to assume the throne. For her alleged actions, Mary was imprisoned in the Tower of London where she eventually lost her head on the chopping block.

When James Stuart was old enough to rule, he was installed on the throne as King James VI. In 1603, the unmarried Queen Elizabeth I died and James VI succeeded her on the English throne, adding the title James I to his name. In 1625, James's son Charles succeeded him on the throne as Charles I. Charles I was a weak leader and was swayed by the influence of the Catholic Church. Charles' weakness and unpopularity eventually resulted in him losing his head on the chopping block in 1649.

With Charles I dead, the rule of England, Scotland, and Wales fell under the authority of a series of parliaments for over a decade. This period of authoritarian rule, known as the interregnum period, featured the influence of puritan Oliver Cromwell. In 1660, when Cromwell died, Charles I son, Charles II, was invited to return from exile to assume the throne. When Charles II died in 1685, his younger brother James assumed the throne as James II. But James II soon came under a cloud of suspicion when he expressed Catholic leanings. In 1688, he was driven from the throne. To save his neck from the executioner's axe, he fled to France with financial help from Louis XIV. James' daughter Mary and her Dutch husband William of Orange then assumed the English throne at the behest of English parliament. With that, the Stuart dynasty ended.

In 1707, the English and Scottish parliaments united to form the Parliament of Great Britain. In 1716, France sought better relations with England, so James was shuffled off to Rome where he lived on a stipend from the French government. Behind the scenes, however, James agitated for a Stuart member to assume the English throne once again and he encouraged rebel groups (Jacobites) in the Scottish Highlands to push back against English rule. While in Rome, James married Maria Sobieski, the grand-daughter of Polish King John III Sobieski. James and Maria had two children – Charles Edward Stuart and Henry Benedict Stuart. Henry went on to become a Roman Catholic cardinal and had little or no interest in any efforts to return a Stuart to the throne of England. Charles, who became known as Bonnie Prince Charlie, became deeply involved in the Jacobite cause. Jacobite forces under Charlie's command won battles at Prestonpans in 1745 and at Falkirk in 1746. The Second Battle of Falkirk was to be the last battle won by Bonnie Prince Charlie and his troops. The next battle would be the devastating Battle of Culloden which forever ended the Jacobite ambitions and the potential for a Stuart to return to the English throne.

FALKIRK'S ECONOMY SHIFTS

As the political monarchy intrigue was unfolding, the economy of Falkirk was developing. In 1600, Falkirk was granted Mercat (market) status. Markets (fairs) were a regular sight in Falkirk. Farmers from across the Scottish highlands, and northern England would congregate in Falkirk to buy and sell animals and produce. With the coming of the railways around 1840, the need to congregate in one place diminished and Falkirk's economy shifted from agriculture to industrial manufacturing.

Coal, limestone, and ironstone deposits were plentiful in the nearby area. These three resources are the key ingredients in iron and their availability soon prompted the manufacturing landscape around Falkirk to have a focus on iron foundries. The success of the foundries was further aided by the ship building industry centered in nearby Glasgow. Long made of timbers, ships hulls were starting to be made of steel. Anchors, anchor chains, porthole windows, rudders, and propellers were also starting to be made of cast iron smelted in local foundries.

Further driving this economic shift was the use of cast iron to manufacture consumer items such as fans, stoves, and even sewing machines. The next time you see an antique pot-bellied cast iron stove, or an old Singer treadle sewing machine, think of the area around Falkirk, Scotland. The black cast iron bodies of the Singer sewing machines were made in the local foundries as were the pot-bellied stoves.

Thanks to the Forth and Clyde canals and to the railways, manufactured goods from the greater Glasgow area could be exported internationally. The late 1800s saw a surge in new foundries as demand for consumer items intensified. In 1899 alone, five new foundry facilities were built in Falkirk. However, this late expansion marked the peak of the market for consumer, cast items. As the 1900s dawned, overcapacity, price competition, and shrinking profit margins began to mark the tenor of the Falkirk economy.

Working conditions in the foundries were less than pleasant. Iron dust defined Falkirk in the early 1900s. The hours were long and the work was hard. Workers suffered from dust inhalation, fever, and a lung disease called blackspit. Despite the dirt and dust, workers were not provided with material for facemasks. Concerns over working conditions stoked organizational sentiment which resulted in the formation of labour unions. Two of the largest unions were the Central Ironfounders Association, and the Associated Society of Ironmoulders.

THOMAS DOUGLAS AND ANNIE CLEMENT

Work in one of the hot, dusty foundries was the daily reality for ironmoulder Thomas Douglas. Work in the cotton mills was the daily reality for Annie Clement and had been since 1895 when she first went to work at the age of sixteen. Clement's family had come from the Scottish highlands so her father, Andrew Clement, could take up a job at the shipping docks in Glasgow. He was Conservative leaning in his political views and Baptist in his faith. History books are not clear as to exactly when Annie and Thomas married.

On October 20, 1904, Annie gave birth to their first child, a son – Tommy Clement Douglas. It could not be envisioned at the time, but this child would go on to have a profound impact on politics several thousand miles away in a place called Saskatchewan.

Thomas and Annie would go on to have two more children – Annie in 1908, and Isabel in 1910.

- The geopolitical threads and historical intrigue woven through Falkirk extend from the executioner's chopping block all the way to Bonnie Prince Charlie.
- In the late 1800s, Falkirk was a focal point for heavy industry, a fervent labour union movement, the Baptist faith, and the politics of change.
- Tommy Douglas was born October 20, 1904 in Falkirk, Scotland and was destined to become a political scrapper like his ancestors.

2

To Canada and a Better Life

CLASS DISTINCTION

As demand for consumer cast items peaked, the Falkirk foundry industry began to experience financial difficulties. Thomas Douglas decided sitting around hoping for better times was pointless. He was disappointed with the class distinctions that pervaded society. The *Poor Law*, dating back to 1601 was at the heart of this class distinction. The *Poor Law* placed blame for poverty at the feet of the lower classes.

He was aware of the scarcity of working-class representation in the British House of Commons. Changing society's problems would require getting involved in politics; not an easy feat for a working-class man. The only way for a working-class person to enter the political sphere would be through pretending to be middle-class – and this is exactly what Scottish union member Kier Hardy pulled off in 1892. He pretended to be middle class, won the confidences of the Liberal Party brass, and ran for office.

His election marked a change in the tide. Working class men now had a voice in Liberal politics.

Hardy soon revealed his background and quickly became the voice in the House of Commons for working class people. The Liberal Party brass were not pleased. But Kier Hardy was not deterred. In 1893, he was elected Chairman of the newly founded Scottish Independent Labour Party. The new Party suffered from a lack of organization and a wide diversity of opinion and platforms. It found itself unable to gain support from the large labour unions; the election of 1895 saw the Party trounced at the polls. What the Party did accomplish, however, was an opening of the door to Labour politics in Scotland. In 1900, labour unions that upheld the socialist ideals of the Scottish Independent Labour Party formed the Labour Representation Committee. Several years later, in 1906, this Committee evolved into the Labour Party. Kier Hardy with his bold effort at pretending to be middle class had changed the face of Scottish politics.

SLOW PROGRESS

By 1909, the Labour Party had managed to influence Liberal Prime Minister Herbert Asquith. In his budget, he stated that *"… four spectres haunt the poor: old age, accident, sickness, and unemployment. We are going to exorcise them."* To provide more social services to lower class people, his budget introduced an income tax of 9 pence per pound on incomes up to 2000 pounds and a 12 pence (1 shilling) per pound tax on incomes above 2000 pounds. Asquith's budget was approved, along with this new tax, in 1910 by King George V.

Watching this slow political progress did not please Thomas Douglas. There was a new country called Canada that was beckoning immigrants. Thomas's younger brother Willie had already been to Canada and back and his descriptions of Winnipeg encouraged Thomas to make the move. Thomas was also no doubt thinking about his son's future in industrial Falkirk. Young Tommy was an active child who enjoyed playing outdoors.

One day he suffered a nasty fall which left a deep gash on his leg. A bone infection, osteomyelitis, set in which began to cause him persistent pain. A local Scottish doctor came to the Douglas residence to examine Tommy's leg. The doctor laid young Tommy on the kitchen table and anaesthetized him. The doctor then scraped the femur of the infected leg. Unfortunately, the treatment proved ineffective at curing the osteomyelitis. Falkirk was no place for a growing lad with a bone infection in his leg. Working in the foundries or in the ship yards demanded physical fitness. Tommy's condition cast a dark shadow over his future in industrial Falkirk.

TO WINNIPEG

The disappointing kitchen table medical effort to help young Tommy propelled Thomas Douglas into action. In 1910, he gathered up his wife Annie and their young children. They answered the beckoning call of Canada and headed for Winnipeg, Manitoba.

A big attraction for immigrant families was the 1908 revisions that had been made to the Dominion Lands Act. Settlers to the western provinces could homestead a quarter of land (160 acres) plus buy a nearby quarter for $3 per acre. But Thomas Douglas was not interested in homesteading. He was attracted to Winnipeg by its strong working-class movement and socialist politics. The family took up residence in the north end of Winnipeg. Thomas secured employment at the nearby Vulcan Iron Works where his prior work experience as an ironmoulder in Falkirk made him an easy hire.

One winter, Tommy's osteomyelitis leg injury flared up. He was able to attend school only because two neighborhood boys pulled him there on a sleigh each day. When his leg situation did not improve, Tommy ended up in hospital. The doctors decided the only solution to the leg infection was to amputate the leg. A stroke of good fortune intervened at the last minute. Dr. Stanley Alwyn Smith, an orthopaedic surgeon at Winnipeg's Children's Hospital, agreed to perform an expensive and complicated corrective procedure for free so long as it could be observed by his medical students. The operation saved Tommy's leg from amputation. Although not realized at the time, this fortunate event also shaped young Tommy's character. Years later, the Province of Saskatchewan, and indeed all of Canada, would be the beneficiary.

WORLD WAR I

A couple years after the family arrived in Winnipeg, the political winds began to shift in Europe. Between late 1912 and early 1913, Greece, Serbia, Montenegro, and Bulgaria joined forces to defeat the Ottoman Empire. Bulgaria, unhappy with its gains from this conflict, turned on its three war partners in June 1913. This effort did not go well and Bulgaria ended up gaining very little from the conflict. Serbia, however, fared well in the conflict, and began flexing its political muscle. An intimidated Austro-Hungarian empire pleaded with Germany for support in the event that a now emboldened Serbia ever moved to attack. The Germans refused to offer support.

Meanwhile, Russia was recovering economically from its 1905 defeat at the hands of the Japanese in the Russo-Japanese war. France made it clear that if conflict broke out between Serbia and Austria-Hungary, the French would support Russia. Germany, sensing that Russia might one day turn unfriendly, reconsidered its position and offered to support Austria-Hungary if conflict were to break out.

On June 28, 1914, Archduke Franz Ferdinand, the heir presumptive to the Austro-Hungarian throne, was assassinated by a radical Serbian student as the royal motorcade drove through the streets of Sarajevo (annexed by the Austro-Hungarian empire in 1908). This gunshot set off a cascade of political events. Weeks later, Austria-Hungary declared war on Serbia. Germany declared war on Russia and France. Britain declared war on Germany. Canada, being a loyal British colony stepped up to support Britain.

In 1914, Thomas Douglas gathered up Annie and the children and returned to Scotland where he enlisted in the Scottish 12th Field Ambulance Brigade. Annie and the children lived in Glasgow with her father while Thomas was away at war. In April 1916, Thomas Douglas transferred from the Ambulance Brigade to join the Canadian Expeditionary Force who offered to pay him $1.10 per day.

In Glasgow, Tommy went to school. To help his mother financially, he worked four hours each weekday and all day on Saturdays in a nearby barber shop. In the summer of 1918, at age 13, he was hired on at a cork factory and was soon promoted, becoming the owner's office assistant. Tommy quit school to work at the factory full-time, earning the handsome sum of three pounds per week.

Glasgow shaped young Tommy's values. When not working, he would often venture across the city to Glasgow Green where he would listen to soapbox speakers criticize and condemn government policy. On Sundays, he would attend the local Baptist church with his mother. Tommy was doing more than just listening and attending. He was observing the structure of the messages, from the soapbox and pulpit alike. He was observing the speech patterns, the voice intonations. He witnessed firsthand the neutralizing impact of a speaker briefly empathizing with those who disagreed with him. He learned how a story could put listeners at ease and soon have them laughing. Although he did not realize it at the time, these skills would one day be on full display when he entered the political arena in Canada. His experiences at Glasgow Green also steeped him in Labour movement politics from firebrand speakers calling for workers to put down their tools and stop supporting the war effort to Liberal speakers like David Lloyd George who spoke of implementing a tax on land owners and aristocrats with the proceeds to be used for social programs.

As 1918 slowly progressed, substantial gains were made by allied troops on the war front lines. On November 9, 1918, German Kaiser Wilhelm

II abdicated and fled to Holland. Two days later, Germany agreed to the Allied terms and signed the armistice. The war was over.

When Thomas Douglas reunited with his family in Glasgow after the armistice, the class distinction theme was still evident in society and he decided that the family should return to Canada. Thomas's earlier decision to transfer to the Canadian Army made the move relatively easy; the Canadian government would pay the cost of moving the family to Winnipeg. In January 1919, Annie and the children boarded a boat in Liverpool and made their way back to Canada. Thomas would follow as soon as his post-war military duties were completed.

The Spanish Flu pandemic broke out in January 1918. In Canada, it killed 55,000 people out of a population of eight million. The worst of the pandemic hit Winnipeg in April 1918. The flu was highly virulent, often killing people within 24 hours. Healthy people in their twenties and thirties were prime candidates for falling ill; they thought themselves to be healthy and refused to observe precautions such as wearing masks. In Winnipeg, out of a population of 180,000, 1,200 people died. By late 1918, the worst of it was over. By not returning to Winnipeg until January 1919, Annie might well have side-stepped exposing herself and her children to the virus.

WHEAT AND THE RAILWAYS

What the Douglas family had also sidestepped with their decision to spend the war years in Glasgow was the economic volatility that hammered the western provinces during the war. But as they were about to realize, the post-war years would be just as volatile.

In 1917, the Canadian government suspended the open market system and assumed monopoly control over grain sales by way of the Board of Grain Supervisors (later named the Canadian Wheat Board). Farmers received an initial payment for their grain followed later in the year by a final payment which was based on the number of bushels grown across the western provinces that season. In 1920, with the war over, the government shut down the Board and reverted back to the open market system. No sooner had the government restored the open market system than the world price of wheat fell sharply in response to Australia and Argentina selling their bumper crops of grain. In 1919, a bushel of western Canadian wheat under the Board of Grain Supervisors system fetched $2.63. By 1923, that same bushel of wheat was selling for 65 cents. Adding to the misery and low prices was an inability for farmers to efficiently get their wheat to market.

In 1917, three railway companies hauled grain to market: Grand Truck Pacific, Canadian Northern, and Canadian Pacific. But in 1919, the Grand Trunk Pacific and Canadian Northern railways declared bankruptcy, leaving only the Canadian Pacific Railway operating.

Canadian Northern Railway traces its origins to Manitoba and the late 1890s. Railway entrepreneurial contractors Sir William Mackenzie and Sir Donald Mann expanded branch lines into the grain growing regions of Manitoba to compete with the Canadian Pacific Railway. Mackenzie and Mann next decided to push eastward. By 1901, the Winnipeg-Port Arthur line was completed which opened a route to get grain to the port at Fort William-Port Arthur (modern day Thunder Bay). Next came a push westward to Edmonton in 1905.

But there was competition. The Grand Trunk Pacific Railway had already come to Edmonton and had pushed west into the Rocky Mountains. In 1910, Canadian Northern started laying track west from Edmonton only to find that the Grand Trunk organization had already laid track on the best route. Canadian Northern had to do extensive blasting and tunneling at a substantial cost in order to get its track laid.

To cover the costs, Canadian Northern borrowed heavily from the Canadian Imperial Bank of Commerce. As blasting and tunneling continued to burn through cash, the accumulated debt put the Canadian Imperial Bank of Commerce in financial jeopardy. The bankers realized there was no way the Canadian Northern Railway could generate enough revenues from hauling western grain to Lake Superior to meet its debt obligations. In 1914, the cost of shipping 100 pounds of grain from Saskatoon to Fort William-Port Arthur was 24 cents. In an effort to squeeze more money from farmers and to appease the CIBC bankers, Canadian Northern started raising its shipping costs. By 1919, their cost of shipping 100 pounds of grain had risen to 38 cents and Canadian Northern Railway was no longer competitive with the cheaper shipping costs offered by Canadian Pacific Railway. The federal government took control of the failed Canadian Northern organization. Had the federal government not acted, the Canadian Imperial Bank of Commerce would likely have failed. Such a failure would have had dire ramifications for the entire country.

The Grand Trunk Pacific operation was not immune to budgetary issues either. It had calculated a cost of laying track through the Rocky Mountains at $60,000 per mile. The actual cost came in closer to $100,000 per mile. As the Grand Trunk operation raised its grain shipping costs, it too lost its ability to compete with the Canadian Pacific Railway. In 1919, the Grand Trunk operation defaulted on its debt payments to the federal government which then took over the company. The assets of the failed Canadian Northern and the failed Grand Trunk companies were merged together into a new entity, the Canadian National Railway (CNR).

The inability for these failed railways to compete with the shipping costs offered by the Canadian Pacific Railway (CPR) rests with a deal made by Prime Minister Laurier in 1897. The CPR had come to Laurier seeking help to finance its push westward through the mountains. Laurier agreed to finance track laying from Lethbridge, Alberta to Nelson, British Columbia provided the CPR offer in perpetuity a grain shipping rate of one-half cent to move one ton of grain one mile; all the way from the west to Fort William-Port Arthur. This was the origin of the "Crow Rate."

If one considers that the distance from Saskatoon to Fort William-Port Arthur is 930 miles, the shipping cost agreed to by the CPR equates to $4.65 per ton (23.25 cents per 100 pounds). For farmers who lived near a grain elevator on the CPR line, this freight rate was far better than the 38-cent figure being charged by the financially strapped competitors. The anger of farmers forced to pay the higher freight rates due to their location near the CPR line soon translated into action.

In 1921, a militant group of angry farmers in Ituna, Saskatchewan formed the Farmers Union of Canada. Not only were these farmers upset with the rising freight costs over the past few years, they believed the Winnipeg Grain Exchange was manipulating prices and grades to avail itself of profits that it stood to make from the export of grain. The Farmers Union of Canada would eventually amalgamate with a political movement called the Farmer Labour Party. This grassroots political upswelling would later have an impact on the career trajectory of Tommy Douglas.

STRIKE!

Winnipeg in 1919 was a different place than it had been in 1910 when the Douglas family had first come to the city. The war was over. The demand for munitions and manufactured goods was receding. Factories were closing. Veterans returning home were desperate for work. Shortages of goods drove prices higher. Rents were higher. Fuel was more expensive. A basket of groceries that had cost $6.49 in 1914 was now $11.

Tommy Douglas watched his parents struggle to make ends meet. His mother, Annie, had managed to secure occasional employment at the nearby Singer Sewing Machine factory. To help support their mother and father, Tommy and his two younger sisters periodically dropped out of school, taking part time jobs to make whatever contribution they could to the family. Tommy would eventually drop out of school permanently to take up a five-year apprenticeship as a printer for the Winnipeg-based agricultural publication *Grain Trade News*.

The situation was especially dire for common construction labourers, who worked a 60-hour week at a wage of 30 cents an hour. In the building trades, the highest paid workers were stone carvers, who earned 87.5 cents an hour for a 44-hour week. On May 1, 1919, Winnipeg's building and metal workers went on strike demanding higher wages. Two weeks later, the Winnipeg Trades and Labour Council sounded the bell for a general strike in support of the metal workers. The response was overwhelming. Soon, over 30,000 union and non-union workers had walked off their jobs. Grain elevators shut down, trams stopped running, and postal and telephone communications came to a halt. Sympathy strikes started breaking out across the country.

Two years earlier, something similar had happened in Petrograd, Russia. Hungry protestors looking for bread had taken to the streets. Supported by huge crowds of striking industrial workers who had lost faith in the leadership of Czar Nicholas, the bread-seeking protesters clashed with police. Military troops were called out to restore order. Troops opened fire and several protestors were killed. A few days later, Czar Nicholas abdicated. A provisional government took the helm, but several months later it was overthrown by leftist Bolsheviks led by Vladimir Lenin.

The Canadian government under Sir Robert Borden feared the Winnipeg events could lead to a similar outcome. Borden's Solicitor General, Arthur Meighen, fanned the flames when he said, "The leaders of the general strike are all revolutionists of varying degrees and types, from crazy idealists to ordinary thieves."

James Shaver Woodsworth, a Winnipeg Protestant minister and social activist who had joined the strikers on the streets, disagreed with Meighen saying "This strike is not engineered from Russia. In reality, the strike has nothing to do with revolution. It is an attempt to meet a very pressing and immediate need. The organized workers – like everyone else– are faced with the high cost of living. Like most people, they imagine that if they can get higher wages, they can buy more food."

The Borden government in Ottawa took swift action; ordering all striking federal employees to return to work immediately or face dismissal. Believing that immigrants were behind the strike effort, the Borden government then amended the Immigration Act so non-British-born immigrants could be deported. The Criminal Code's definition of sedition (incitement to rebellion) was broadened to afford Borden more power to tamp down on the dissent.

Meanwhile, the mayor of Winnipeg, Charles Gray, fired most of the city police force on the basis that he felt many officers were sympathetic to the strikers. He replaced the fired constabulary with 1,800 special constables, recruited and paid for by the business community. The special constables each received a horse and a baseball bat with which to keep order. The North West Mounted Police (NWMP) were also brought in. On June 10, 1919, a riot broke out after the special constables tried to disperse a crowd listening to a speech. A few days later, the federal government arrested twelve union leaders, forbade the publication of the *Western Labour News,* and ordered the NWMP to put down demonstrations using any necessary force.

On June 21, 1919, war veterans organized a parade to protest the restrictions and a crowd of 6,000 people gathered in front of City Hall. A streetcar operated by strikebreakers approaching City Hall drew attention from the veterans who then overturned it and set it on fire. With that, the NWMP and the special constables charged the crowd.

Editor of the *Western Labour News,* Fred Dixon wrote: *Then with revolvers drawn, the Mounted Police galloped down Main Street, turned, and charged right into the crowd on William Avenue, firing as they charged. One man, standing on the sidewalk, thought the Mounties were firing blank cartridges until a spectator standing beside him dropped with a bullet through his breast. Dismounted red coats lined up and declared military control.*

This event, as memorialized in the screenplay *Strike* and its sister movie

Stand!, resulted in two strikers being killed, thirty-four others wounded, and the police making 94 arrests. Fearing more violence, workers decided to call off the strike. On June 25, at exactly 11:00 in the morning, the strikers returned to work. Forty days after it began, the largest social revolt in Canadian history had been crushed. Seven of the arrested strike leaders were convicted of a conspiracy to overthrow the government and sentenced to jail terms ranging from six months to two years. Protestant minister James Shaver Woodsworth was arrested and charged with writing newspaper editorials critical of government authorities, though he was never convicted.

One of the part-time jobs Tommy had, was delivering newspapers. It was while on his delivery route on June 21 that the noise and commotion on William Street caught his attention. For safety, he scrambled up the fire escape ladder on a building to take refuge on the rooftop. As he watched the action below, a young Tommy Douglas saw NWMP officers fire into a crowd of striking workers. Bloody Saturday, the violent end of the Winnipeg General Strike; two men shot dead; the family's pastor J.S. Woodsworth arrested. These events would forever shape the ideals of Tommy Clement Douglas.

- When Tommy Douglas was five years old, a playground accident left a gash on his leg. Pain from a subsequent bone infection, osteomyelitis, would be with him for the rest of his life.
- When Tommy Douglas was faced with the prospect of having his leg amputated, an orthopaedic surgeon agreed to perform surgery on the leg at no charge to the family. This fortunate event shaped young Tommy's views of the medical system.
- In 1910, the Douglas family left Scotland for prospects of a better life in Winnipeg, Manitoba. When World War I broke out, the Douglas family returned to Glasgow, Scotland so

that Tommy's father could serve with the Scottish 12th Field Ambulance Brigade.

- Young Tommy would often visit Glasgow Green to listen to soapbox speakers criticize and condemn government policy. On Sundays, he would attend the local Baptist church with his mother. Tommy was doing more than just listening and attending. He was observing the structure of the messages, from the soapbox and pulpit alike. He was becoming steeped in Labour party politics. His character was being shaped.

- Following the war, the family returned to Winnipeg. Tommy took on various part-time jobs to help support the family. One of these jobs was delivering Saturday papers. One Saturday in 1919, while on his delivery route, he witnessed NWMP officers fire into a crowd of striking workers. This event, Bloody Saturday, marked the violent end of the Winnipeg General Strike. What Tommy Douglas saw that day would forever shape his ideals.

3

Religious Studies

In the aftermath of the 1919 events, Tommy began to take an interest in the Baptist religion, no doubt inspired by the Sunday sermons at the Baptist church in Glasgow and his maternal grandfather's affiliation with the Baptist church. Before long, Tommy was using his spare time to give talks at a local Baptist church and helping out as a part-time preacher. He joined a youth fraternal group run by the Freemasons called the Order of DeMolay. He found he enjoyed opportunities at DeMolay meetings to recite prose that members were required to memorize and recite. A member of the Freemasons Lodge noticed his talent for oratory and convinced him that he should consider attending university after finishing his five-year printing apprenticeship.

Even though he was of small stature, Tommy had an interest in boxing. When not involved with church or DeMolay activities, he could be found around the boxing ring at One Big Union gym. He was fast on his feet and quickly developed his skills in the lightweight boxing category. He went on to win the lightweight championship of Manitoba in 1922 and again in 1923. However, there was no career to be had in boxing and after his 1923 win, he hung up his boxing gloves and resolved to become a full-time Baptist preacher.

In the fall of 1924, at the age of 20, Tommy Douglas enrolled at Brandon College where he would spend the next six years. Brandon College, founded in 1899, was funded by Baptist Churches across western Canada. The mandate of the college was to graduate Baptist ministers with a skill for critical thinking and analysis. The first three years at Brandon College were focused on completing the high-school education he had skipped while working at his printing apprenticeship to help support his family. The next three years were focused on the religious study required to become a Baptist minister.

He paid his way through college by filling in as a relief preacher in towns and villages in rural Manitoba, mainly in the summers. Economic times were tough and many rural congregations could not afford a full-time preacher. One of the congregations he was sent to was the village of Austin, Manitoba, not far from Brandon. The church was slated to close and Tommy was to deliver the last few sermons and then wind down the church. Instead, he challenged the congregation. He urged them to get out into the surrounding area and recruit new members. He even traveled around the countryside on a bicycle, visiting rural families who might join. This rural experience gave him considerable insight into the cares, concerns, culture and psychology of rural people. The experience of rallying a group of people to take up a cause would serve him well in his political future.

The 1920s were a highly charged time within the Baptist faith, and indeed within the Methodist and Presbyterian faiths as well. Biological and geological discoveries around the world were challenging the Biblical story of creation. In 1859, Charles Darwin had published his theory of evolution in a book entitled *On the Origin of Species by Means of Natural Selection*. Darwin's ideas for decades afterwards were the stuff of academic debate. Initially, his ideas were not discussed by individuals outside of academia. But as the 1920s dawned, discussion of evolution spilled over into mainstream discourse and into the church pulpit. So intense was the controversy, major Protestant groups in North America suffered a serious divide. On one side of the wedge, modern, progressive congregations favoured bringing new scientific theory into the pulpit. On the other side of the wedge, evangelical fundamentalist congregations fought to keep scientific thinking out of the pulpit. One of the more famous examples of this wedge divide played out in the United States. The *Scopes Monkey Trial* reached its climax in a Dayton, Tennessee courtroom where high school teacher John T. Scopes had been charged by the State of Tennessee for having violated statute law by teaching Darwinian evolution in his classroom.

At Brandon College, similar controversy between Baptist progressives and Baptist fundamentalists was on full display. Creationism versus Darwinian science was a hotly debated issue. Should the Baptist faith concern itself with personal salvation and the after-life? Or, should it focus on Social *Gospel*, the applying of Christ's message to solving everyday social problems? As the storm of controversy swirled, Tommy Douglas was caught right in the middle. His experiences over the next couple years in the classroom would have a lasting effect on his view of the world.

Tommy's professors generally supported the doctrine of *Social Gospel*. They said that Christian ethics and morals should be applied to issues such as poverty, alcoholism, crime, racial tensions, slums, unclean environment, child labour, lack of unionization, poor schools, economic inequality, and the dangers of war.

As Tommy became steeped in this way of thinking, he began to realize these were the very issues that had shaped his father's decision to leave the iron foundry in Falkirk, Scotland to seek a better life in Canada. Tommy became aware of the limits of the fundamentalist beliefs that many Baptist congregations were still holding fast to.

Tommy was highly influenced by Harris Lachlan MacNeill – his professor of Greek and Latin and acting Dean of the College. MacNeill was the author of *The Christology of the Epistle to the Hebrews* which rejected literalist, fundamentalist interpretations of the Bible. MacNeill became so mired in fierce debate with the fundamentalist wing of the college that he was accused of heresy. Although the allegations were ultimately withdrawn, the experience had badly shaken both the faculty and the students. MacNeill's views would stick with Tommy, who became fond of comparing the Bible to a double bass fiddle, in the sense that "you can play any tune you want on it."

In later life when Tommy reflected on MacNeill, he said, "He took the position that the Bible was a library made up of poems like the Psalms, drama like the Book of Job and the Book of Esther, historical books, letters such as the Epistles of St. Paul, prophecies, and actual biographical accounts like the Gospels. He thought that each of these should be interpreted in light of the purpose for which they were written."

Another firebrand professor that Tommy was influenced by was Professor Buttenhard who taught a socialism economics course with emphasis on Marxist theory. The knowledge gleaned from this course further shaped the ideals of Tommy Douglas.

In Tommy's final year (1930) at Brandon College, he was asked, along with classmate Stanley Knowles, to provide weekend relief preaching duties at Calvary Baptist Church in Weyburn, Saskatchewan. Tommy had considerable experience as a relief preacher in rural Manitoba, and he quickly impressed the congregation in Weyburn with his down-to-earth style and sense of humour. After graduation, he was asked to become the congregation's pastor. Knowles ended up at First Baptist Church in Winnipeg. The career paths of these two men would cross again many years later in the House of Commons in Ottawa.

- At the age of 20, Tommy Douglas enrolled at Brandon College where he completed his high-school education as well as the religious study needed to become a Baptist minister. He paid his way through college by filling in as a relief preacher in towns and villages in rural Manitoba.
- One of the congregations he was sent to was slated to close. Instead of accepting this fate, he challenged the congregation to find new members and save the church. His rural experiences gave him considerable insight into the cares, concerns, and psychology of rural people.
- The 1920s were a highly charged time within the Baptist faith. Creationism versus Darwinian science was being hotly debated. In the US, the Scopes Monkey Trial was driving a wedge between Baptist progressives and Baptist fundamentalists. At Brandon College, similar controversy raged between faculty members.
- Tommy Douglas decided to reject the literalist, fundamentalist interpretations of the Bible. He decided to focus on applying Christian ethics and morals to issues such as economic inequality, living conditions, labour issues and unionization.

4

Marriage and Weyburn, Saskatchewan

IRMA

During his time at Brandon College, one of Tommy's Sunday relief-preaching assignments took him to Carberry, Manitoba. It was there that he first laid eyes on the charming Irma Dempsey. Soon after, they became reacquainted when she began attending Brandon College as a music student. One day, they found themselves on opposing sides of a resolution in a debating event. Tommy and his team lost the debate, but he gained a companion. They married in the summer of 1930 – he was 25 years old and she was 19. The couple would go on to have two daughters: Shirley Jean, born in 1934, and Joan, whom they adopted in 1945.

SHIRLEY

Young Shirley inherited her father's skills for oration and performing. She also inherited his penchant for social justice. Shirley's acting career began in 1950 with a role in the Regina Little Theatre's entry at the

Dominion Drama Festival in Calgary where she won the best actress award. The Dominion Drama Festival was an annual event, held each year in a different Canadian city. Its aim was to promote amateur theatre. In 1952, Shirley graduated from the Royal Academy of Dramatic Art in London. She stayed in England for several years, performing for theatre and television. In 1957, she returned to Canada and married Timothy Sick whose father owned Sick Brewery in Lethbridge, Alberta. Shortly after, she gave birth to a son, Thomas. The marriage ultimately did not work and the couple divorced.

Her travels then took her to Italy where she did voice dubbing on spaghetti western movies. It was on one of these ventures that she met Canadian actor Donald Sutherland. In 1966, Shirley and Donald married. She soon gave birth to twins, Rachel and Kiefer. In 1967, she and Donald and the three children moved to Los Angeles, California. While Donald pursued his acting career, Shirley became involved in the American civil rights movement. She joined campaigns to speak against the Vietnam War, and lobbied on behalf of immigrants and women. She perhaps pushed her advocacy too far when she helped establish the fundraising group "Friends of the Black Panthers". In 1969, she was arrested in Los Angeles for Conspiracy to Possess Unregistered Explosives. According to a sworn statement by FBI agents, she allegedly attempted to purchase hand grenades for the Black Panthers from undercover FBI agents. In defense, she claimed the FBI framed her by creating a crime where none existed prior to their involvement. Subsequently, the US government denied her a work permit based on this allegation against the FBI. Having divorced Donald Sutherland, and unable to secure a work permit, she and her three children left America in 1977 and moved to Toronto where she pursued an acting career. She passed away in 2020 at the age of 86.

WEYBURN

In the summer of 1930, Tommy Douglas took up his ministry duties in Weyburn, Saskatchewan. Weyburn traces its history to 1892 when the railway laid an extension line from Brandon. One year later, the Soo Line from the US Border arrived. Being at the intersection of two railways helped the tiny settlement grow quickly. A post office was opened in 1895 and a land office was opened in 1899 to assist the settlers who were starting to arrive. The community grew so fast that it became a village in 1900, a town in 1903, and a city in 1913.

Topographically, Weyburn is situated in the semi-arid "Palliser Triangle"named after John Palliser, a former Captain in the British militia. Palliser became intrigued with the prairies during an 1847 hunting expedition which moved him to write *Solitary Rambles and Adventures of a Hunter in the Prairies*. Between 1857 and 1861, he spent more time on the prairies as the leader of the British North American Exploring Expedition. During 1857 and 1858, the expedition party travelled over what is present day Saskatchewan, cataloguing the local flora, fauna, and minerals. Palliser identified a large, triangular region that he believed was unsuitable due to its general shortage of rainfall and lack of timber. This region, now formally called the *Palliser Triangle*, runs diagonally from west of Kindersley to near Estevan and is bounded by the US border to the south.

Palliser's 1857-58 observations eventually rang true. The general shortage of rainfall coupled with homesteading settlers turning sod on the virgin prairie seriously upset the ecosystem in the Palliser Triangle region. By the 1930s, the shortage of annual rain soon turned into a complete absence of rain as local weather patterns shifted due to the changed ecosystem. Adding to the stresses of homesteading farmers was the North American economy being mired in depression following the collapse of stock market between 1929 and 1932. Wheat prices were low, money was scarce, farm families were devastated. Federal government inspectors would visit families at their homes to administer a "means test". People would have to remove their shirts so the inspector could see their ribs. If their ribs were clearly visible, some meagre federal government assistance would be provided.

NOT YOUR TYPICAL PREACHER

Instead of just an impersonal, biblical sermon from the pulpit on a Sunday morning, Tommy Douglas opted for some levity with such topics as "Jesus and Capitalism" and "Jesus and War." He also opted for more traditional practices, such as prayer meetings and revivals, that met the spiritual needs of his parishioners. Tommy's progressive leanings instilled in him by his professors at Brandon College compelled him to go beyond just preaching about charity. He decided to offer charity. He and Irma worked tirelessly to get clothes and food shipped in for the desperate farm families in the Weyburn area. His church's basement soon filled with donations, which they then distributed to the needy; even if those people did not belong to his Weyburn congregation.

THE PROGRESSIVE MOVEMENT

Tommy devoted what spare time he had to furthering his studies. In 1933, he was granted his Master of Arts degree in Sociology from Brandon Collage. Brandon College had gained its degree-granting authority by virtue of its affiliation with McMaster University in Hamilton, Ontario. Part of his degree studies required completing a thesis project. His thesis research would take him back into the swirling controversy between the progressive and the evangelical fundamentalist wings of the Baptist Church. The academic debate stimulated by the 1859 release of Darwin's book eventually led to the question of whether it would be possible for mankind to selectively breed better quality humans by focusing on their heredity traits. This line of thinking earned the label, *eugenics*. One of the more notable figures to have embraced eugenics early on was Winston Churchill, who in 1912 infamously said, "multiplication of the feeble minded is a terrible danger to the race."

Teaching of eugenics spread like wildfire across North America. In 1928 alone, 376 college courses in the United States were dedicated to the subject of eugenics. Eugenics also filtered through into Canadian politics. In 1921, the Saskatchewan government in cooperation with the Canadian government established the Weyburn Mental Hospital, in part to segregate individuals who did not fit into society. In Alberta in 1928, the government passed the *Sexual Sterilization Act.*

Another luminary who embraced eugenics was American economist Irving Fisher, who is known for his contributions to monetary theory and reserve banking theory. He co-founded the American Eugenics Society, which was soon accompanied by the American Race Betterment Society and a publication called the *American Breeders Magazine.* Irving Fisher is unapologetically remembered both as an economist and a eugenicist. Such was the Progressive era of the 1920s.

After discussions with his advisors at McMaster University, a program of research was agreed upon that would take Tommy Douglas into the Weyburn Mental Hospital to gather data. His thesis was entitled *The Problems of the Subnormal Family* and it openly endorsed the concept of eugenics.

His thesis research focused on twelve prolifically reproductive, "mentally subnormal" women, some of whom resided at the Weyburn Mental Hospital. These twelve women had given birth to a total of 95 children, who in turn had given birth to children of their own. His research found that of the 95 children, 34 had become moral delinquents. A total of 34 moral delinquents from twelve mentally subnormal women led Douglas in his thesis to propose a system that would require couples seeking to marry to be certified as mentally and morally fit. He made the argument that those deemed to be "subnormal" because of low intelligence, moral laxity, or venereal disease should be segregated from the general population and sent to government institutions. Moreover, he made the argument that mental defectives and moral delinquents should be sterilized.

- In the summer of 1930, Tommy Douglas took up his ministry duties in the town of Weyburn, Saskatchewan.
- In addition to his pulpit duties, he and his wife worked tirelessly in charitable efforts to collect donations of clothes and food, which they then distributed to people in need, including many who did not belong to his Weyburn congregation.
- In 1933, he was granted his Master of Arts degree in Sociology from Brandon Collage. His thesis paper, entitled *The Problems of the Subnormal Family*, took him back into the swirling controversy over Charles Darwin's 1859 query as to whether it would be possible for mankind to selectively breed better quality humans by focusing on their heredity traits – *eugenics*.

5

A Changed Man

THE COAL MINER'S STRIKE

In the late 1850s, Palliser's expedition had noted coal seams along the Souris River but decided they were of little economic value. A few decades later, as the CPR and the Soo Line came through the area, local farmers seeking to mine small bits of coal to sell to the railways realized that the coal seams were more extensive than Palliser had realized. In 1896, the Souris Valley Coal Company opened a commercial coal mine. In 1906, the Canadian Pacific Railroad (CPR) opened Bienfait Mines Ltd. to obtain lignite coal for its steam locomotives. The various mines flourished, but the miners working at the mining operations did not. As more profits were extracted by the mining companies, the conditions of the miners became worse with many mine workers being fatally injured on the job.

The coal seams were wet. To mitigate the wetness, the mines operated in the winter when the moisture in the seams was frozen. To compensate for only working in the winter months, the mine workers put in 80 hours per week. Even with the wet coal seams frozen, working conditions were plain miserable. The coal seams in the area were up to 60 feet beneath the surface. To access the seams, a sloped tunnel would be excavated from surface down to the coal seam. The coal was shoveled by hand, and manually hoisted into small rail trolley cars. The loaded trolley cars would then be pulled out of the mine, back to the surface. Forty tons a day of coal was the average production for a man.

Those who couldn't find any other work during the summer shutdown bought their food on credit at the company store. In the winter, when they went back working at the mines, their bills were deducted from their earnings. Frequently discrepancies arose concerning dollar amounts on the bills, but so desperate were these men for work that they dared not challenge the company. In the aftermath of the 1929 financial market collapse, the price of coal dropped; layoffs became common; working conditions worsened. Something had to change. And it soon did.

Saskatchewan was not the only province with shallow coal seams. Parts of Alberta had similar geology. Working conditions in the Alberta coalfields were every bit as arduous as in Saskatchewan. In the 1920s, coal workers in Alberta embraced the United Mine Workers of Canada union movement and began demanding higher wages and better working conditions. As working conditions worsened in the Saskatchewan coal mines, the union organizers in Alberta took notice.

In August 1931, with help from Alberta organizers, a committee representing nearly 600 local coal workers established the first Saskatchewan local of the United Mine Workers of Canada. The new union local immediately demanded a wage increase, an end to the company store model, better living conditions, and improved workplace safety. Management at the local mining operations refused to recognize the union as legitimate and refused their demands. Management regarded the union movement as being associated with Soviet Russia. Management was emboldened in its attitude thanks to Section 98 of the Criminal Code of Canada. This amendment and its provision for a five-year jail term had been added to the Criminal Code in 1919 by the Borden government as a means of suppressing radical activity and preventing working class challenges to the established order of society.

On September 7, 1931, the unionized coal miners voted to go on strike. Union leaders called for a general work stoppage. On September 18, Tommy Douglas publicly spoke to a group of the miners, telling the story of Moses leading the Israelites out of Egypt with the Pharoah in pursuit. He explained that the Israelites had no choice but to go forward. He encouraged the miners to make the slogan "go forward" their rallying cry. In his Sunday sermon two days later (entitled *Jesus the Revolutionist*) he asked his congregation, "Would Jesus revolt against our present system of graft and exploitation? How would Jesus view the coal miners' strike?" He organized a supply of food for the miners and their families, an action that may have soured some of the more pro-business members of his congregation.

On September 29, 1931, a group of miners, along with their families, assembled in Estevan to parade through the city in order to draw attention to their strike. Upon entering the Estevan town square, the miners were confronted by the RCMP. Violence broke out, the RCMP opened fire on the strikers, killing three strikers of Ukrainian heritage and injuring numerous others. The following morning, 90 RCMP officers raided the miners' homes. Strikers and union leaders were arrested on charges of rioting. The RCMP involved with the killing of the miners were not charged. In their report to Ottawa, the local RCMP command described how the unionized workers had been carrying red flags and had been armed with clubs. The report claimed the strikers had opened fire first.

In light of the tragic violence, on October 6, 1931, the mining company conceded to key demands including a $4 minimum wage, an 8-hour working day, reduced rent, and an end to the company store practices. A victory, yes. But at a substantial cost. It was later learned that Prime

Minister Bennett had ordered the Department of Immigration and Colonization to deport mine workers who were non-naturalized immigrants, who had been convicted of vagrancy, or who had applied for public assistance. Anti-immigrant sentiment was deeply embedded in corporate management and in Ottawa politics.

TO CHICAGO FOR PH.D. STUDIES

Troubled by the events in Estevan, Tommy Douglas decided to pursue further education. In the summer of 1933, he turned his attention to getting a Ph.D degree from the University of Chicago. While doing his field research, he became deeply disturbed by the hobo camps around Chicago where he saw nearly 75,000 transients in make-shift shelters surviving by begging or stealing on the streets. Douglas interviewed despondent men who had once belonged to the American middle class - bank clerks, lawyers and doctors. He observed soup kitchens run by the Salvation Army and local churches and how, in the first half-hour of the day, their food offerings were cleaned out. Those that did not receive food spent the rest of their day begging on the streets of Chicago. He was left with a feeling of hopelessness. He was equally disturbed that members of the Socialist Party sat around quoting Marx and Lenin, waiting for a revolution to occur, while refusing to help the destitute. Douglas is reported to have said, "I've no patience with people who want to sit back and talk about a blueprint for society and do nothing about it." Although elected political office was not yet on his mind, this profound statement would one day come to define the actions of Tommy Douglas when he became Premier of Saskatchewan.

Abandoning his Ph.D studies, Tommy Douglas returned to Weyburn with a very different outlook on life. He was changed as a person. Not only had his Chicago experience affected him, so too had the events surrounding the 1931 Weyburn Miner's Strike.

- In the late 1850s, the Palliser expedition noted lignite coal seams along the Souris River. Years later, the Soo and CPR rail lines coming through the area created a market for mining this coal. The various mines flourished, but the miners' working conditions did not.

- In August 1931, nearly 600 local coal workers established the first Saskatchewan local of the United Mine Workers of Canada. The newly unionized coal miners voted to go on strike. After marching on Estevan, the miners were confronted by the RCMP who opened fire, killing three strikers and injuring numerous others. The following morning, RCMP officers raided the miners' homes. Strikers and union leaders were arrested on charges of rioting.

- In 1933, Douglas turned his attention to getting a Ph.D. degree from the University of Chicago. In the hobo camps around Chicago, he saw nearly 75,000 transients living in make-shift shelters, surviving by begging or stealing on the streets of Chicago.

- The miner's strike and the Chicago hobo camps changed Tommy Douglas. He is reported to have said, "I've no patience with people who want to sit back and talk about a blueprint for society and do nothing about it." Although elected political office was not yet on his mind, this profound statement would one day come to define Tommy Douglas when he became Premier of Saskatchewan.

6

Saskatchewan Politics in 1929

The Saskatchewan election of 1929 saw Liberal Premier James (Jimmy) Gardiner ousted. Gardiner (MLA for Melville,) had been Premier since 1926 but had come under fire for alleged patronage appointments. His stance towards the Klu Klux Klan also worked against him.

After the votes were counted, the Conservatives under James Thomas Milton Anderson (MLA for Saskatoon) had in theory won, taking 28 seats to the Liberal's 24 seats. The Progressive Party took 5 seats, and Independent candidates 4 seats. In an aggressive move to prevent Anderson from being sworn in as Premier, Gardiner reached out to these nine fringe MLAs and put together an agreement for a minority coalition government. The Lieutenant Governor accepted the minority coalition plan and Gardiner was again sworn in as Premier. However, the fledgling government soon fell apart and was defeated in a motion of non-confidence. Instead of having another election, the Lieutenant Governor asked Anderson to form a coalition government.

Even though Gardiner was no longer the Premier, his heavy-handed influence continued to play a role in what happened in Saskatchewan. He enjoyed solid connections to the owners of radio stations and newspapers in the province. He had connections that ran deep into the ranks of law enforcement. Gardiner's sphere of influence was known as the "Gardiner Machine". Even the events that unfolded a few years later in 1931 in Estevan had the Gardiner Machine fingerprints on them.

As well as concerns over patronage appointments, Gardiner's failure to win a majority in the 1929 election was tied to his sentiment over the Klu Klux Klan. As University of Saskatchewan graduate student Gordon Unger describes in his 1967 MA thesis paper, the origins of the Klan trace back to the post-Civil-War period in America. The Klan was opposed to having federal money spent on rebuilding the war-torn South. The Klan fomented for anti-Negro violence. Eventually, though, it lost popularity and faded in influence (but never disappeared entirely) as the US government advanced its policy of rebuilding the South. Seeking to revive itself in the 1920s, the Klan began to again promote its anti-immigrant position using cross burnings, lynchings, beatings, and even murders to drive home its philosophy. The Klan realized that Canada held substantial promise for new membership and expansion of activity. A membership drive in Toronto in 1925 attracted 700 new, paid members in one month alone.

The Klan grew so rapidly it became a victim of its own success. In 1927, disagreements among top members saw the movement split into two factions. One of these factions turned its sights on western Canada; Saskatchewan in particular. The province in 1927 was financially stable, which helped the Klan in selling new memberships. The homesteaders in Saskatchewan were mainly immigrants who had held on to their old-world customs and practices. As well, an undercurrent of anti-Catholic sentiment was flowing strong in the province. Saskatchewan was the perfect recipe for advancement of the Klan. Premier Gardiner was aware of the Klan's movement towards Saskatchewan and hired detectives to investigate Klan activity in Toronto and in several American cities. As Gardiner was busy investigating, the Klan was busy marketing. Before long, the Klan had sold a reported 13,000 memberships in Saskatchewan priced at $13 each. But then…the money disappeared.

In the fall of 1927, Gardiner attacked. He ridiculed the Klan and pointed to how they had just stolen $169,000 from hard-working Saskatchewan people. In January 1928, Gardiner took his stance into the Legislature, delivering a well-detailed summary of Klan activity and going so far as to suggest the opposition Conservative party was linked to the Klan. One of the Klansmen thought to have stolen the $169,000 was American activist Pat Emmons. When he disappeared to the USA (allegedly with the money), he offered to help Indiana authorities quell the Klan movement in that state in exchange for avoiding prosecution. Emmons then returned to Canada and, in a series of carefully orchestrated speeches, suggested that he had proof of Conservative Party involvement with the Klan. With the Klan exposed as a money-stealing entity and with the Conservatives in uproar, Gardiner concluded that he had done enough on the Klan issue to ensure his political future and turned his attention to the next election.

But Gardiner had miscalculated. Although the Klan as an organization was wounded in status, it had stirred up considerable emotion among Protestant voters across the province. The Conservatives fanned the flames of unease towards immigrants that the Klan had promoted. The Conservatives promised greater control over future immigration to Saskatchewan and even went so far as to suggest a policy of compulsory English education for all immigrant children. Moreover, the Conservatives played on rumours that the federal government was planning to bring 100,000 French-speaking, Catholic settlers into the province. Gardiner could not stem the tide of unease and came up short in his effort to remain Premier. Even an attempt at forming a coalition government came up short.

The Klan very much wanted a Protestant, white, province of Saskatchewan.

Now, as Leader of the Opposition, Gardiner revived his efforts to use the Klan as a political tool. He regularly accused Premier Anderson's Conservative government of having links to the Klu Klux Klan. The 1930s were tough economic times for prairie homesteaders, many of them immigrants. The last they wanted to hear about was a political party with an anti-French, anti-Catholic, anti-immigrant, pro-British, Klan viewpoint.

Gardiner kept the pressure on Anderson's Conservative government. This was a unique time in Saskatchewan politics. Never before had there been such a large number of MLAs on the Opposition side of the chamber. Gardiner and his team knew where to find information and statistics. They knew what questions to ask during legislative sittings. Gardiner and his MLAs kept the Anderson government tied up in knots. Gardiner was determined to regain his status as Premier in the next election.

When the next election came in July 1934, Gardiner defeated Anderson to again become Premier. Gardiner's Liberals took 50 seats and the CCF took 5 seats. Anderson and his Conservatives were shut out completely and the Gardiner Machine was back in control. These five CCF seats would soon prove to be something of a proverbial acorn from which a mighty tree would grow.

GARDINER GOES TO OTTAWA

Having clawed his way back into power and once again into the role of Premier, Jimmy Gardiner started looking for new challenges. One of his first moves was to eliminate the Saskatchewan provincial police force that the previous government had created and bring the RCMP back to police the province. Gardiner also mistrusted bureaucrats, especially those over which he had no control. The Anderson coalition had created the Public Service Commission which hired bureaucrats on the basis of their merit and granted them significant autonomy. Gardiner swiftly abolished the Commission, hiring bureaucrats whom he knew and could control.

He took his reforms one step further and abolished the provincial Relief Commission. Granting of relief payments to people in need was now controlled by his Cabinet.

Despite his heavy-handed approach to politics, Gardiner did have some threads of compassion. In 1928, he had passed a piece of legislation called the *Saskatchewan Sanitoria and Hospitals Act*, designed to provide free hospitalization and treatment for victims of tuberculosis. Gardiner also pressed hard for Ottawa to relinquish its grip on resources. He felt that the mineral and oil resources of Saskatchewan belonged to the people of Saskatchewan. Gardiner was also a proponent of government ownership of power and telephones. In 1928, the Gardiner government passed the legislation to bring the Saskatchewan Power Commission (known as Sask Power today) into being.

The re-elected Gardiner government of 1934 soon found itself swept up in social unrest. Canada was locked in the grip of the Dirty Thirties depression. Commodity prices had fallen; exports had plummeted, and on the prairies, drought had set in. To counter the depression, Conservative Prime Minister Bennett allocated $20 million for shovel-ready, public works projects. To avoid communist sentiment riling up the masses of unemployed across the country, Bennett created relief camps administered by the Defense Department. In June 1935, nearly 1,000 hungry, desperate men walked away from a relief camp in Vancouver and jumped on eastbound railcars. They decided to make the trek to Ottawa to confront the Bennett regime. Bennett and his Ministers decided to watch in amusement; there was no way these men riding in box cars would ever make it to Ottawa.

When the rail cars started rolling across Saskatchewan, heading for Regina, Bennett and his team began to panic. Prime Minister Bennett was well aware of Jimmy Gardiner and the Liberal politics that had unfolded in the province. Bennett instructed the RCMP to intervene when the trains arrived in Regina. Gardiner protested. He warned Bennett that trying to intervene would cause a riot. Bennett seemed not to care. He had no political affiliation with Gardiner, nor did he like him as a person. On July 1, 1935, a public rally assembled in downtown Regina in support of the trekkers. When the RCMP started to break up the rally, all hell broke loose between police, trekkers, and residents of Regina. Guns were drawn. Shots were fired. At the end of the fracas, two people were dead, hundreds were wounded, and thousands of dollars of damage had been done.

The outcome was not what Bennett had hoped for. To defend his government, he was now faced with the prospect of calling a general election. His own Party was badly divided over how the economy had been handled. Voters were unhappy as well. William Lyon McKenzie King and his Liberals promised more effective action in stimulating the economy. When the votes were counted, King was the new Prime Minister. His Party had taken 173 seats and the Bennett Conservatives only 39. There was a newcomer on the Opposition side of the Commons—long-time friend of Tommy Douglas, Winnipeg preacher, turned CCF politician, J.S. Woodsworth, whose Party had taken 7 seats.

The On-to-Ottawa Trek disaster in Regina was hardly what Gardiner had been hoping for either. He knew that the events of the Regina riot would dog him in the Legislature. He needed new challenges; new opportunities. He did not have to look too far. In November 1935, Prime Minister King offered Gardiner the position of Minister of Agriculture using the emoluments clause provision in the 1867 Constitution Act. Gardiner stepped down as Premier, turning the task over to Deputy Premier, William Patterson. King then made arrangements for Gardiner to run in a federal by-election in January 1936 in south-east Saskatchewan in the riding of Assiniboia. Gardiner handily defeated the CCF candidate 7,282 to 3,717 votes.

Jimmy Gardiner was off to Ottawa. He would hold the agriculture portfolio for the next 22 years, until the Liberals were defeated in the 1957 federal election by Saskatchewan's own John Diefenbaker.

- In the 1920s, the US-based Klu Klux Klan promoted its anti-immigrant position in western Canada.
- Premier Jimmy Gardiner was a harsh critic of the Klan and used his criticism as a platform for the 1929 election. But the Klan had stirred up considerable emotion among Protestant voters across the province who were not about to vote for a Premier who opposed the Klan. The Gardiner Liberals were defeated.
- As Leader of the Opposition, Gardiner used the Klan as a political tool, accusing the ruling Conservatives of having strong Klan connections. The 1930s were tough economic times for prairie homesteaders, many of them immigrants. The last they wanted to hear about was a political party with an anti-immigrant, pro-British, Klan viewpoint.
- The 1934 election saw the Gardiner Liberals returned to power. The new Gardiner government soon found itself swept up in the social unrest of Canada being locked in the grip of the Dirty Thirties depression.
- In June 1935, nearly 1000 hungry, desperate men walked away from a relief camp in Vancouver and jumped on eastbound railcars. When the railcars reached Regina, the RCMP moved to break up a public support rally. Guns were drawn, shots were fired. Two people were dead, hundreds were wounded, and thousands of dollars of damage had been done.
- To defend his government, Prime Minister Bennet called a general election. William Lyon McKenzie King and his Liberals promised more effective action in stimulating the depressed economy and were voted into office.
- Prime Minister King offered Gardiner the position of Minister of Agriculture. Gardiner stepped down as Premier, ran in a federal by-election in south-east Saskatchewan in the riding of Assiniboia and went on to hold the agriculture portfolio for the next 22 years.

7

Render Unto Caesar

At Brandon Collage, Tommy Douglas had studied the economics of socialism, guilds, communism, and capitalism, but purely from an academic standpoint. Now, in light of his Chicago hobo camp experience, his MA degree thesis research, and his striking coal miner experience, he began to ask himself "what is wrong with the economic system? Why is it so dysfunctional? "

Many in his Weyburn congregation were asking similar questions. People had taken the economic system for granted, assuming it would be there to help when help was required. Yet, Tommy Douglas was seeing a whole generation of young people facing poverty, misery, and lack of opportunity. He concluded that practicing charity by distributing donated goods and clothing was no longer sufficient.

He decided to take more direct action. He established a labour exchange in Weyburn that allowed people who were short of cash to get day jobs by offering up whatever marketable skills they had. He created a club to provide boys from poor families with direction, encouragement, and hope, even teaching the boys basic boxing skills. He helped organize the Weyburn Independent Labour Association in an effort to pressure political leaders to create a program of unemployment insurance. He spoke out in favor of equal rights of all citizens, and public ownership of basic utilities.

It soon became obvious to Douglas that in order to do more for society he would have to step down from the pulpit and enter the political arena. The transition would be an abrupt one. Baptist Church policy at the time said that there was no place in the church for politics. God and politics did not mix. Church policy further stated that a minister could not so much as run for political office and stand in the pulpit at the same time.

Despite these policies, Douglas arranged a meeting with Secretary Balsom of the National Baptist Council. When he raised the possibility of running for political office while still preaching, Secretary Balsom reminded Douglas of Jesus' words: *render unto Caesar the things which are Caesar's.* In other words, leave politics alone and focus on preaching.

This answer was not good enough for Douglas. He began to speak out on Sundays when he took to the pulpit. The social gospel philosophy that he had subscribed to at Brandon College rose to the surface. One Sunday, he told the story of one of his wife's relatives in Manitoba who had a sick child. The local hospital wanted cash to admit the child. The family could not find the money; the child died. The hospital was a legal entity, it had every right to demand cash payments up front. But how did the actions of this hospital align with the premise of "love thy God and love thy neighbour?"

Seeing people all around enduring poverty and misery, he began to speak out against the church's dogmatic positions. He argued that it was time for a new interpretation of Christianity. It was time for young people to build a better society rather than live in misery clinging to the hope of gaining some uncertain Biblical reward in the dim, distant future.

Douglas had an ally in his political leanings. A local parishioner couple, Charlie and Lally Lawson, were involved in an upstart political party called the Farmer Labour Party (FLP). This Party had come about in 1932 after the Farmers Union of Canada and the Independent Labour Party had merged with the United Farmers of Canada Party (Saskatchewan section). Charlie and Lally encouraged Douglas to get more involved in this new movement.

Major James Coldwell had been chosen to lead the new Party. (Major was his first name, not a military title). Major Coldwell had been born in Seaton, England on December 2, 1888. After attending Exeter University, he left England in 1910 to become a school teacher in the village of New Norway, Alberta (near present day Camrose, Alberta). He returned to the United Kingdom during his 1912 summer break and married Norah Gertrude Dunsford whose father was a wealthy newspaper owner. The couple moved to Canada, where he continued teaching; this time in Sedley, Saskatchewan where he eventually became involved with politics.

In 1932, delegates from the various farmer-led political Parties traveled to Calgary for a convention designed to unite the parties as well as labour groups from western Canada. What emerged from this convention of unification was a new party called the Cooperative Commonwealth Federation party (CCF).

In addition to Coldwell, a key figure that had emerged on the political scene was Clarence Fines. Born August 16, 1905, in Darlingford, Manitoba, Fines took his education at the University of Manitoba and the University of Saskatchewan. After graduation, he became a school teacher. One of his first teaching assignments was in Sedley, Saskatchewan where he met Major Coldwell. Fines' view of the political landscape agreed with Coldwell's and soon Fines was actively involved in politics. He chaired the 1932 Calgary convention that gave rise to the CCF.

Thatcher versus Douglas

- In light of the coal miners' strike and his Chicago experience, Tommy Douglas began to wonder what was wrong with the economic system? Why was it so dysfunctional?
- Despite warnings from the National Baptist Council, Tommy Douglas began to let politics slip into his Sunday messages from the pulpit.
- Two parishioners, Charlie and Lally Lawson, were involved in an upstart political party called the Farmer Labour Party (FLP) and encouraged Tommy Douglas to get more involved in this new movement.
- In 1932, delegates from the various farmer-led political Parties met in Calgary and created a new party called the Cooperative Commonwealth Federation party (CCF).

8

The Regina Manifesto

In the summer of 1933, the CCF Party held its first convention in Regina. A figure from Tommy Douglas' past, Winnipeg minister James Shaver Woodsworth, was elected as the leader of the party. The official Party platform adopted at this convention was called the *Regina Manifesto*.

The CCF Party agreed it would work towards a co-operative mindset in Canada. The goal behind the production, distribution, and trade of goods would become one of satisfying human needs, not one of making profits.

The CCF Party further agreed it would work towards eliminating class distinction and class exploitation. Waste, instability, insecurity, and inequality would also be eliminated. The extremes of feverish prosperity and catastrophic depression were due to financiers and industrialists and their focus on profit. Extreme economic swings would be removed through a planned and socialized economy where resources, production, and distribution were controlled by the people.

The CCF Party promised to promote individuality and the rights of racial groups and religious minorities.

The CCF platform believed that the old political Parties in Canada were controlled by capitalist interests and were not capable of social reform. The CCF party would campaign hard to get its candidates elected so as to begin economic transformation.

The following is a summary of what the fourteen parts of the Regina Manifesto called for:

1. **Planning**

    A National Planning Commission will be established to ensure the efficient functioning of the economy and to co-ordinate the activities of socialized industries. The commission will be staffed by public servants.

2. **Socialization of Finance**

    Banking currency, credit, and insurance will come under government control. The chartered banks will be socialized and removed from the control of private, profit-seeking interests. A Central Bank will be established to control the flow of credit and general prices, and to regulate foreign exchange operations. A National Investment Board will direct unused surplus goods to more socially desired purposes. Insurance companies, which charge needlessly high premiums for the services that they render, will also be socialized.

3. **Social Ownership**

    Transportation, communications, electric power and all other industries and services essential to social planning will be socialized. This includes entities at the national, provincial, and municipal levels. Public utilities will be operated for the public benefit; not for private profit. Natural resources will be developed in a like manner. Mining, pulp and paper-and even the distribution of milk, bread, coal and gasoline-will be brought under social ownership and operation.

The welfare of the community must take supremacy over private wealth. A CCF government will not play the role of rescuing bankrupt private concerns for the benefit of promoters and stock and bond holders. The management of publicly owned enterprises will be through boards of people appointed for their competence in industry. Rigid Civil Service rules will be avoided as will patronage appointments.

Workers in public industries will be free to organize into trade unions and will be given the right to participate in the management of the industry.

4. **Agriculture**

The security of tenure for a farmer should be laid down by individual provinces. Farmers should be provided with insurance against crop failure. Tariff burdens on agricultural products should be removed. The efficiency of exporting farm products should be enhanced. Internal price levels (floor prices) should be raised so that the farmers' purchasing power is restored.

The intense depression in agriculture today is a consequence of the general world crisis caused by the capitalistic system resulting in: (1) economic nationalism expressing itself in tariff barriers and other restrictions of world trade; (2) the decreased purchasing power of unemployed and under-employed workers and of the Canadian people in general; (3) the exploitation of both primary producers and consumers by monopolistic corporations who absorb a great proportion of the selling price of farm products.

Agricultural depression has resulted in the catastrophic fall in the world prices of foodstuffs as compared with other prices; this fall being due in large measure to the deflation of currency and credit. To counteract the worst effect of this, the internal price level should be raised so that the farmers' purchasing power may be restored.

The position of the farmer should be improved by: (a) more cooperatives being created for the purchase of farm supplies and domestic requirements; and (b) more cooperatives created for the processing and marketing of farm products.

5. **External Trade**

   External trade should be managed through import and export boards. Canada can only acquire external supplies if she exports goods produced. The strangling of export trade by insane protectionist policies must be brought to an end. Canada must organize the buying and selling of her main imports and exports under public boards, and take steps to regulate the flow of less important commodities by a system of licenses.

6. **Co-operative Institutions**

   Cooperative enterprises should be assisted by the state through appropriate legislation and through the provision of adequate credit facilities.

7. **Labour Code**

   A National Labour Code should be created (through BNA Act modification) to help workers maximize income and leisure. Insurance covering accident, old age, and unemployment should be offered. Workers must have freedom of association and be given participation in the management of industry.

   Technological developments have made possible a high standard of living for everyone. There must be a reduction of the hours of work in accordance with technological development and a constantly rising standard of life for everyone who is willing to work. The Labour Code must include state regulation of all wages, equal reward for equal services, irrespective of sex; a right to work provision, the right to unemployment insurance, social insurance to protect workers against the hazards of sickness, death, industrial accident and old age, limitation of hours of work, and protection of health and safety in industry.

Workers must be guaranteed the right to freedom of association, and should be encouraged and assisted by the state to organize themselves in trade unions. By means of collective agreements, workers can achieve fair working rules and share in the control of industry and profession.

8. Socialized Health Services

A healthy population should be the responsibility of every civilized community. Health services should be made freely available. A system of public health services, including medical and dental care, that stresses the prevention rather than the cure of illness should be provided to all people in both rural and urban areas.

9. B.N.A. Act

Amendments to the B.N.A. Act should be obtained to ensure that the existing rights of racial and religious minorities are not be changed without their own consent. The present division of powers between Dominion and Provinces reflects the conditions of the 1867 pioneer era. The constitution must be brought into line to reflect the industrialization of the country and the centralization of economic and financial power.

The Canadian Senate has developed into a haven of capitalist interests, as illustrated by the large number of company directorships held by its aged members. The model of a fixed number of members appointed for life is an obstacle to be abolished.

10. External Relations

A Foreign Policy should be designed to obtain international economic cooperation and to promote disarmament and world peace. Genuine international cooperation is incompatible with the capitalist regime in force in most countries. The League of Nations has evolved into the League of Capitalist Great Powers. Canada should stand against participation in imperialist wars. Canada must refuse to be entangled in any more wars fought to make the world safe for capitalism.

11. Taxation and Public Finance

Capitalist governments in Canada raise a large proportion of their revenues from customs duties and sales taxes on consumer goods; the burden of which falls upon the masses. In place of such taxes, we propose a drastic extension of income, corporation and inheritance taxes, steeply graduated according to ability to pay.

The capitalist system relies on public debt creation. All public debts have enormously increased, and the fixed interest charges now amount to the largest single item of public expenditures. The CCF proposes that in future no public financing shall be permitted. Capital shall be provided through the National Investment Board and shall be free from interest charges. The exception will be Public Works projects which shall be financed by the issuance of credit in alignment with the National Wealth of Canada (GDP).

12. Freedom

The CCF Party believes in freedom of speech and assembly for all. Section 98 of the Criminal Code (preventing the joining of unlawful associations, passed in 1919 after the Winnipeg Strike) should be abolished. The Immigration Act should be amended to prevent deportation. Equal treatment before the law of all residents of Canada irrespective of race, nationality or religious or political beliefs should be offered.

13. Social Justice

The CCF Party promotes the establishment of a commission composed of psychiatrists, psychologists, socially minded jurists and social workers, to deal with all matters pertaining to crime and punishment so as to humanize the law and to bring it into harmony with the needs of the people.

14. An Emergency Program

The Dominion Government must directly deal with the critical unemployment situation by a program of public spending on housing, and other enterprises to be financed by the issue of credit based on the National wealth. Unemployed workers must be secure in the tenure of their homes, and the scale and methods of relief must be such as to preserve decent human standards of living.

It is recognized that even after a Cooperative Commonwealth Federation government has come into power, a certain period of time must elapse before the planned economy can be fully worked out. During this brief transitional period, we propose to provide work to those who are unemployed by a program of public expenditure on housing, slum clearance, hospitals, libraries, schools, community halls, parks, recreational projects, reforestation, rural electrification, elimination of grade crossings, and other similar projects in both town and country. This program, which would be financed by the issuance of credit based on the national wealth, would serve to create employment and meet social needs. This program must include guarantees of adequate wages and reasonable hours of work, and must work towards a Cooperative Commonwealth.

The present depression is a sign of the mortal sickness of the capitalist system. This sickness cannot be cured by the application of salves which leave untouched the cancer which is eating at the heart of our society, namely, the economic system in which our natural resources and our principal means of production and distribution are owned, controlled and operated for the private profit of a small proportion of our population.

No CCF Government will rest content until it has eradicated capitalism and put into operation the full program of socialized planning which will lead to the establishment in Canada of the Cooperative Commonwealth.

Douglas was not involved in crafting the wording of the Manifesto. In fact, he felt the wording was perhaps too restrictive, especially with its call for eradication of capitalism. He felt this wording could restrict the CCF Party from election wins. Nevertheless, he decided to press ahead on a foray into the political sphere.

- In 1933, the CCF Party held its convention in Regina. The official Party platform adopted at this convention was called the *Regina Manifesto.*
- It called for a more efficient economy, government control of banking and essential services, more help for farmers, a National Labour Code, and free health services, among other things.
- Tommy Douglas was feeling the pull of politics. It was time to test the political waters.

9

Provincial Candidate
T.C. Douglas

Douglas approached Coldwell and Fines to express his interest in being the CCF candidate for the riding of Weyburn in the 1934 provincial election. They both reminded him that the CCF was a new creation and that getting elected amidst the power of the Gardiner Machine would be difficult.

Undeterred, Douglas decided to run. He took to the pulpit one last time and announced to his congregation that he would be stepping down as their pastor to run for political office.

Coldwell and Fines advised him to divide the Weyburn riding into zones and to get volunteers to help in each zone. Douglas and his volunteers devised a strategy of distributing CCF Party literature to immigrant families in the riding written in their native languages: Ukrainian, Russian, and German.

Despite the hard work by the Douglas campaign, this strategy of reaching out to immigrant families was not enough. Gardiner had countered the CCF platform by suggesting to immigrant homesteaders that the CCF would expropriate all their farmland, just like the Communist Party had done in the Soviet Union. Additionally, Gardiner's war against the Klan had highlighted the issue of immigration. Protestant, non-immigrant voters were concerned about the waves of immigration coming into Saskatchewan. Voters concerned over an issue tend to show up at the polling stations to cast their ballot.

In the Weyburn riding, Douglas came in third, well back of the winning Liberal candidate Hugh Eaglesham and just behind the Conservative incumbent, Presbyterian minister Robert Leslie. Liberal candidate Eaglesham got 2,281 votes, defeated incumbent Leslie got 1,544 votes, and Douglas 1,343 votes. At the party level, the CCF took five seats and the Gardiner Liberals the remaining 50 seats.

For a new upstart Party, taking 10% of the seats in the Legislature was a good start. The momentum would only keep growing in the years to come.

- Tommy Douglas let his name stand as the CCF candidate for the riding of Weyburn in the 1934 provincial election.
- Despite the hard work and excellent organization by the Douglas campaign, the Gardiner machine countered the CCF platform by suggesting to immigrant homesteaders that the CCF would expropriate all their farmland, just like the Communist Party had done in the Soviet Union.
- After the votes were counted, Douglas finished in third place.

10

Federal Candidate
T.C. Douglas

Undeterred by his 1934 defeat in the provincial riding of Weyburn, Douglas turned his sights to the coming 1935 federal election. Perhaps his boxing experience played a role here. Despite his recent provincial election defeat, Douglas was still standing. He was still in the fight. He could go another round.

The Prime Minister was R.B. Bennett. Originally from New Brunswick, Bennett had studied Law at Dalhousie University in Halifax before heading west to Calgary in 1897. He established a law firm in Calgary and soon realized vast sums of money, not only from practicing law but from well-timed investments in the new province of Alberta. Financially comfortable, in 1911 Bennett turned his focus to federal politics. Representing the riding of Calgary West, he served as Minister of Justice in Arthur Meighen's Conservative government of 1920-1921. Despite losing his seat by a meagre 13 votes to upstart Canadian Labour Party candidate Joseph Shaw in the 1921 federal election, the voters of Calgary West returned Bennett to Ottawa in the 1925 election.

CRISIS IN OTTAWA

In the October 1925 election, Meighen's Conservative Party took 115 seats. William Lyon Mackenzie King's Liberals took 100 seats and the Progressive Party took 22 seats. Suddenly the country lurched headlong into a constitutional crisis. Meighen did not have enough seats to form a majority. King, thanks to some backroom dealmaking, reached a pact with the Progressives and announced that he could form a coalition government. But King had lost his own seat in the Ontario riding of York North and could not sit in the House of Commons. The day after the election, King went to the Governor General, Lord Byng, who advised, "There are three alternatives as I see it. The first is dissolution, that I hope you will not ask for, and that I would not wish to grant at this stage because the people do not want another election immediately. The next is that Mr. Meighen, having the largest solid group of seats, be called on to form government and the third that you should continue. I shall of course agree to whatever you say as to the last two, but Mr. King, as a friend of yours, may I say that I hope you will consider very carefully the wisdom of the second course."

Instead of opting for the Governor General's second approach of letting the Meighen Conservatives form a minority government, King decided to pursue governance with his fledgling Liberal-Progressive coalition. King would take a seat in the visitor's gallery in the House of Commons and watch the proceedings. To keep the coalition functioning, King agreed to work towards implementing Old Age Security and to lowering taxes. Meanwhile, behind the scenes, the political wheels were turning. The MP for the Saskatchewan riding of Prince Albert, former pharmacist Charles McDonald, agreed to resign his seat. A by-election was triggered, and in February 1926, King sailed to a lobsided victory over the Independent candidate. With that, Mr. King took his chair once again in the House of Commons.

But scandal was about to erupt. Jacques Bureau, the Minister of Customs and Excise, had been fingered in a bribe-taking scandal. In exchange for political favours, Bureau had been receiving liquor on which excise duties had not been paid and his personal driver had received a car. To remove Bureau from the spotlight, King quickly elevated him to the Senate. But it was too late. The House of Commons was in an uproar. King went to the Governor General seeking a dissolution of parliament and the calling of a general election. But Lord Byng refused. In protest, King resigned his seat in the House of Commons. Lord Byng offered the Meighen Conservatives a chance to form a coalition, which they did. The Liberals, minus their leader, argued that Lord Byng was a representative of a foreign power that was influencing Canadian politics. A series of non-confidence motions then followed, the fifth of which took down the Meighen government. A general election was called for September 1926.

King again ran in the Prince Albert, Saskatchewan riding where he handily defeated the Conservative candidate, a young lawyer by the name of John Diefenbaker. Nationally, the Liberals came away with 116 sets, the Conservatives 91 and the Progressives only 11.

Prime Minister Bennett

The events of 1925-1926 proved too much for Arthur Meighen. With King's Liberals now in a majority position, he resigned the Conservative Party's leadership. R.B. Bennett was elected to replace the outgoing Meighen and so became leader of the Opposition.

Bennett would soon have his chance at being Prime Minister. In 1930, Prime Minister King called an election. The stock markets had collapsed in 1929 and the economy was showing signs of slowing dramatically. The heady days of the 1920s were now over. Voters were not happy; the King Liberals were shown the exit, and the Bennett Conservatives were elected with 135 seats. The Liberals took 89 seats, the United Farmers 9 seats, and the Progressives 3 seats.

However, Bennett's governing skills left something to be desired. He claimed to be a supporter of *Imperial Preference Trade Policy* with Britain. An Imperial Preference Trade Policy is based on the principle of home producers first, empire producers second, and foreign producers last. However, Bennett was unable to work with Britain to establish such a policy. He then tried unsuccessfully to copy the New Deal framework that President Roosevelt had implemented in the USA. Bennett promised a fairer taxation system, a maximum work week, a minimum wage, unemployment insurance, workplace accident insurance, changes to the old-age pension program, and support for farmers.

King's Liberals losing power in the 1930 election turned out to be a benefit to the Party. King and his MPs watched as the brunt of the economic slowdown fell squarely on the shoulders of the struggling Bennett Conservatives and their various promises.

STILL STANDING

Douglas' experience campaigning in the 1934 provincial election had fired him up. He was now unafraid to say what was on his mind—that the economic order was unjust and broken. He criticized capitalism and the established political parties; he even went so far as to voice the opinion that churches were supporting the unfair economic system.

Douglas decided to run as the CCF candidate for the riding of Weyburn in the federal election slated for October, 1935. Having seen the On-to-Ottawa Trek take shape and having seen the mess that transpired in Regina, he sensed that there would be a political shakeup in Ottawa.

Before making the formal commitment of running, he had one final talk with Secretary Balsom of the National Baptist Council to fully explore his options. Balsom told Douglas that if he did not stay out of politics, he would never get another preaching assignment, ever again, anywhere in

Canada. Douglas apparently told the Balsom, "You've just given the CCF a candidate."

Douglas wasted little time mobilizing his volunteers from his failed 1934 provincial campaign run. This time, he decided to double down on his oratory skills. He crafted a story designed to resonate with the voter which reminded the voter that there was no benefit in electing one of the other established political Parties. The story was called *Mouseland*.

In Mouseland, every four years there was an election. The mice, time and again, elected a government of black cats. The cats were nice, but they passed legislation that favored cats. They enacted laws that were good for cats. Mouse holes had to be a certain size, to accommodate a cat's paw. The speed of mice was regulated to match the speed of a cat. When it eventually got to the point where the mice could no longer handle this corruption, they voted in another government; this one made of white cats. They even at one point tried a coalition government of half black cats and half white cats. It seems no matter what the mice tried they always elected a government of cats. One day a little mouse asked why could the mice not elect a government of mice? The cats accused that little mouse of being a Bolshevik and locked him up in jail. The mice, taking note of what had just happened, agreed with the idea of electing a government of mice. The mice settled on one profound idea: you can lock up a mouse, you can lock up a man, but you cannot lock up an idea.

The Mouseland fable started to have an impact. Douglas realized this when he started getting his car tires slashed, and when police showed up at his rallies unannounced to disperse the crowds. The Liberal incumbent candidate Douglas was up against was local farmer E.J. Young. Douglas challenged Young to a debate, anyplace, anytime. He then goaded Young by asking him if he was afraid.

This debate challenge highlights an aspect of Tommy Douglas that speaks to his oratory skills and his confidence. This bravado would again be seen in Mossbank, Saskatchewan in 1957.

E.J. Young was campaigning on a platform of protecting farmers by ensuring a better standard of living for them. At the debate, Douglas let Young speak, all while patiently waiting for his turn to pounce. And pounce he did. Douglas had come prepared. He unveiled a copy of the House of Commons' *Hansard* from February 9, 1933. In the Commons on that day, Young had given a speech suggesting quite the opposite of his platform on taking care of the farmer. Douglas distributed copies of Young's Hansard remarks around the room, causing substantial embarrassment for Young who claimed he should not be held accountable for what he had said in the House of Commons. When the votes were counted on October 13 1935, Douglas had 7,280 votes, Young had 6,979, the Communist Party candidate 1,577, and the Social Credit candidate 362. A whiff of controversy lingered in the election aftermath. Douglas had hinted in some of his speeches as to the virtues of the Social Credit Party, which had recently formed government in Alberta. The platform of the Alberta Social Credit movement was one of government intervention in the form of debt-free money given directly to consumers or to producers who sold their products below cost to consumers. What could not be quantified was whether or not any of Douglas' 7,280 votes had come from voters with a Social Credit mindset. The uproar eventually died down and T.C. Douglas, MP for Weyburn, headed for Ottawa.

KING RETURNS TO THE PRIME MINISTER'S OFFICE

The Bennett government suffered a landslide defeat in the 1935 election. King's Liberals were returned to power with 173 seats. The Conservatives limped in with 39 seats. The Social Credit Party took 17 seats, the CCF Party under J.S. Woodsworth took 7 seats, and the remaining 6 seats were taken by a collection of independent parties. Bennett remained leader of the Conservative Party until 1938, when he retired to England. Despite his difficulties in steering the country through the depressed years of the early 1930s, Bennett's legacy does include the creation of the Bank of Canada and the creation of the Canadian Broadcasting Corporation (CBC). However, on a darker note, his story also includes the Regina Riot.

ONE DAY THEY SHALL MEET

At this point, it is interesting to stop for a moment and draw a comparison. It was 1935. Tommy Douglas had educated himself with two University degrees, proven himself a capable Baptist pastor in Weyburn, a powerful orator, a tireless worker on the campaign trail and was headed to Ottawa as an MP. Meanwhile, young Ross Thatcher, who had grown up helping his father run a group of hardware stores in Saskatchewan, had just graduated from Queen's University. He was about to start his first job, a position with Canada Packers in Toronto. As divergent as their paths seemed to be in 1935, their paths were on a course for intersection.

- Undeterred by his 1934 provincial election defeat, Douglas turned his sights to the coming 1935 federal election, letting his name stand as the CCF candidate for the riding of Weyburn.
- The National Baptist Council advised that if he did not stay out of politics, he would never get another preaching assignment, ever again, anywhere in Canada. Tommy Douglas was motivated like never before.
- He mobilized his volunteers from his failed provincial campaign run of 1934. He doubled down on his oratory skills and crafted *Mouseland*, a story designed to resonate with voters by reminding them there was no benefit in electing a government of cats when the mice were perfectly capable of forming government.
- The incumbent Liberal candidate was no match for Douglas. After the votes were counted, T.C. Douglas was headed for Ottawa as the CCF Party MP for the riding of Weyburn.

11

To Ottawa and the
House of Commons

With only a handful of MPs, there was little the CCF Party could do to sway King's Liberals. But Douglas soon drew attention to himself for his speaking ability. He took great delight in aiming barbs across the aisle at the MP from Melville, Saskatchewan, Agriculture Minister Jimmy Gardiner. Douglas used his speaking opportunities in the House to focus on issues related to western farm families and also on Canada's foreign affairs policies. He argued that MacKenzie King's Liberals were doing an inadequate job of dealing with the effects of the Depression. Grain prices were down from the previous two crop years and per-acre yields of wheat, barley, and oats were down due to weather. Farmers had been enduring drought conditions which had created ideal conditions for infestations of wheat stem sawflies, cutworms, and grasshoppers. The coming winter of 1935-36 would prove to be one of the coldest since 1899. The summer of 1936 would mark the peak of the recent drought with temperatures in communities southeast of Regina hitting 45°C.

In the House of Commons, at session after session, Douglas argued the government should act to save family farms by promoting legislation that would encourage land reclamation and water conservation. He argued that the government should act to support grain prices while preventing banks and municipal governments from repossessing land on which farmers had fallen behind on taxes or loan payments. These arguments would soon enough also be heard echoing through the Legislature in Regina.

In addition to the gloomy outlook for farmers, dark storm clouds were also forming in Europe. Douglas brought his concerns to the House of Commons. He argued that the King government should take a stronger position against the aggression of dictators like Italy's Benito Mussolini, and Germany's Adolf Hitler. In 1936, Douglas attended the World Youth Congress meetings in Geneva. He also visited Germany to gauge the impact that the Nazi government was having on the country. He rounded off his trip by visiting Spain where Hitler was helping General Francisco Franco's rebels overthrow Spain's government.

Douglas returned home ready to argue even louder for action by the King government. But CCF Party leader Woodsworth would have none of it. The CCF platform endorsed a pacifist approach. To avoid a full-on fight with Woodsworth, Douglas focused on urging the King government to prevent Canadian companies from selling armaments to Mussolini, Hitler, Franco, as well as Japan.

Douglas was proven right in his assessment when Hitler invaded Poland on September 1, 1939. Having grown up listening to his father's wartime experiences, Douglas detested war but he called for Canada to get ready to fight. This caused another disagreement with Party leader Woodsworth. This disagreement was vocal enough that it created a rift within the CCF Party. Fellow MP, Major Coldwell was watching the rift. Coldwell was onside with Douglas and against the pacifist approach of Woodsworth.

After Canada declared war against Germany on September 10, 1939, Douglas enlisted as a corporal with the 2nd Battalion of the South

Saskatchewan Regiment. He volunteered for active service overseas with the Winnipeg Grenadiers, but was rejected on account of his old osteomyelitis leg issue.

At odds with the CCF Party and rejected for military service he was not giving up. He was still in the fight. He could go another round. This time the boxing ring would be in Saskatchewan.

- In the House of Commons, Douglas argued the government should act to save family farms, support grain prices, and prevent farmland from being repossessing when farmers fell behind on payments.
- As the prospect for war in Europe grew, Douglas argued that the King government should take a stronger position against dictators like Italy's Benito Mussolini, and Germany's Adolf Hitler.
- However, the CCF platform endorsed a pacifist approach. Douglas was now at odds with his own Party. A serious rift was forming between himself and Party leadership.

12

Saskatchewan Beckons

GEORGE WILLIAMS

George Williams was born in November 1894 in the village of Binscarth, Manitoba (not far from Russell, Manitoba). After serving in World War I, he attended the Manitoba Agricultural College and upon graduating in 1920, took a position in Saskatchewan with the *Soldier Settlement Board.*

This Board had been set up in 1917 by the federal government to give financial assistance to any man who had served in the war effort and who was seeking to become established in farming. Applicants for loan assistance were investigated as to their fitness, moral character, assets, and farming aptitude. Loans were made at 5% interest. Loans for animals and equipment were repayable in six annual instalments and loans for land and buildings were repayable in 25 instalments.

In 1921, Williams began farming at Semans, Saskatchewan (between Raymore and Nokomis). He also became involved in politics. In the 1934 provincial election, Williams was elected on the CCF ticket in the riding of Wadena. CCF Party secretary, Major Coldwell, was unsuccessful in getting elected in a Rosetown area riding. However, Coldwell ran federally in the 1935 election and was elected. When Coldwell was elected to the House of Commons in 1935, he resigned the Party secretary position as he headed for Ottawa. Williams became leader of the provincial CCF Party and its four other MLAs. He remained Party leader until 1941 when he enlisted to go overseas.

Williams' decision to enlist to fight overseas left the CCF Party with a leadership vacuum. Major Coldwell and Clarence Fines reached out to Douglas in Ottawa. Douglas easily bowed to pressure from Fines and Coldwell and let his name stand for president of the Saskatchewan CCF Party. Clarence Fines was chosen as Party vice-president. In July 1942, with George Williams still serving overseas, Douglas won the leadership of the Party.

A NEW LEADER

Even though he had been elected leader of the Saskatchewan CCF Party, Douglas continued on in Ottawa as the MP for Weyburn. Clarence Fines earnestly got to work across Saskatchewan building the party base, creating a policy platform, and assembling a team of volunteers. When the House of Commons was not in session, Douglas would come back to Saskatchewan to assist Fines. The two men travelled the province in all directions giving speeches and taking jabs at William Patterson's Liberal government. By April 1944, Douglas and Fines had increased the CCF Party's membership to 26,000.

WILLIAM PATTERSON 1938

William Patterson was born in Grenfell, Saskatchewan on May 13, 1886, a son of Scottish immigrants. He was elected as a Liberal to the Saskatchewan Legislature in 1921. He quickly made an impression on Jimmy Gardiner and soon found himself holding various Cabinet positions. In 1935, when Jimmy Gardiner left the Legislature and the Premier's position to take up a seat in the House of Commons, Patterson was elected Party leader and thereby became Premier.

With the Depression still lingering, Patterson increased funding to assist local school districts that had been defaulting on wages owed to teachers. To raise funds, his government introduced a provincial sales tax with funds raised going directly to the school districts. His government also enacted pension and debt relief legislation, increased labour standards, and expanded funding for the treatment of tuberculosis, cancer, and polio. His government passed legislation making it easier to form credit unions and worker's unions. However, Patterson was of the mindset that deficit spending would ruin the province's credit and refused to run a budget deficit. His position was that government was not Santa Claus and that everyone must pay their share of costs. This mindset did not resonate well with the opposition CCF Party.

Although Patterson railed against the CCF Party and the dangers he felt it posed to democracy, he believed that where a monopoly situation presented itself, government should impose regulation in the best interests of the public. He felt private enterprise could not be relied upon to manage monopoly situations. In the 1938 provincial election, the Patterson Liberals were returned to power, but not with their previous 50 seats. The Liberals took 38 seats, the Social Credit Party two seats, and the Unity Party two seats. The CCF gained five seats to now have 10 MLA's sitting in Regina.

THE CCF PLATFORM 1943

Fines and Douglas unveiled the CCF Party platform in late 1943. There were four components to the platform:

- protecting the rights of farmers to security of land and the rights of workers to organize unions

- expanding the welfare state to include a complete system of socialized health services
- reforming the education system
- building the economy through planning and targeted public ownership.

The Patterson Liberals had just passed the *Legislative Assembly Extension Act*. The Act provided for postponing what should have been a 1943 provincial election into 1944.

Aware of the concerns that the CCF Manifesto had triggered in 1932, Tommy Douglas decided to take advantage of this postponed election to clarify the CCF platform. He made a series of radio broadcasts across the province. He opted for radio so that he could control the narrative. He felt that if he engaged in newspaper interviews, the paper editors, still potentially under the spell of the old Gardiner Machine, would put an anti-CCF spin on any printed articles. In an inspired moment reminiscent of the Mouseland fable, Tommy Douglas created the *Cream Separator* fable to resonate with radio listeners. The following is the text of the fable:

Last week, we discussed the fact that the present economic system would lead inevitably to another worldwide depression after the war. Tonight, I want to suggest an alternative economic system to the one we have at present. I have often likened our present capitalist economy to a cream separator. The farmer pours in the milk — he is the primary producer without whom society would collapse. Then there is the worker — he turns the handle of the cream separator — and it doesn't matter whether he is a coal miner, a railroader, or a storekeeper, it is his labour which makes our economy function. However, there is another person in the picture — he is the capitalist who owns the separator machine. And because he owns it, the machine is run exclusively for his benefit — that is why it is called the "capitalist" system. The capitalist doesn't put in any milk, nor does he turn the handle. He merely sits on a little stool with the cream spout fixed firmly in his mouth while the farmer and the worker can only drink from the skim milk spout. Of course, you can stay alive on skim milk — you will not get very fat, but you will at least be able to live — providing the skim milk keeps on coming; but it doesn't. Periodically the capitalist gets so full of cream that he has indigestion, so he shuts off the machine, which means that the skim milk stops too. When he feels that he can use some more cream, the capitalist starts up the machine again and for a little while he gets the cream and farmer and worker get skim milk. That has been the story of capitalism ever since Canada became a nation. We have a period of prosperity during which the capitalist gets cream and the farmer and worker get skim milk. What then follows is a depression during which the machine does not turn and nobody gets anything, not even skim milk.

THE LIBERAL PLATFORM

The Liberals also released their platform of four points:

- agricultural markets at profitable prices
- protection against the hazards of Nature
- conservation of soil and moisture
- independent ownership and operation of farms.

Patterson especially focused on the fourth point, reminding farmers that farm ownership would be imperiled by a CCF socialist government.

THE 1944 CAMPAIGN

As 1944 dawned, Tommy Douglas shifted his sights back to Saskatchewan. He was the leader of the Saskatchewan CCF Party; he just needed to win a seat in the Legislature. He resigned his position as Member of Parliament in Ottawa and returned to Saskatchewan where he let his name stand in the Weyburn riding.

Douglas campaigned on the dangers of the Liberal Red Menace. The slogan often heard at rallies was *Forward with the CCF*. Douglas campaigned on ten promises:

- Home quarter protection for farm families
- Debt reduction (the province was $178 million in debt)
- Increasing Old Age Pension
- Healthcare reforms
- Larger, more efficient school districts and equal opportunity for people to seek an education
- Increasing Mother's Allowance
- Freedom of speech and religion
- Right to collective bargaining
- More pay for teachers and nurses
- Promotion of co-operatives and sharing of wealth

As the campaign unfolded, the Liberal Party began to lose its appeal to rural voters thanks to its refusal to carry a budget deficit, its sales tax policy, and the idea that everyone must pay their fair share.

TOMMY DOUGLAS M.P. BECOMES PREMIER TOMMY DOUGLAS

On June 15, 1944, Douglas was confident of a CCF victory. The *Regina Leader-Post,* loyal to Premier Patterson's Liberals, was predicting a Liberal triumph. A Gallup poll on the other hand was suggesting a CCF win. What nobody saw coming was a Liberal trouncing. The CCF took 47 of the 52 seats in the Legislature along with 53% per cent of the popular vote. Tommy Douglas, age 39, was now Tommy Douglas MLA and Premier of Saskatchewan.

In Ottawa, Mackenzie King took notice. Historians reading his diary have found comments expressing concern that the socialist CCF might gain power in other provinces and even threaten the Liberal stronghold on Ottawa.

Jimmy Gardiner did not take the news of a CCF win well. He met with Tommy Douglas shortly after the election and suggested subtly that

Douglas should just sit back and allow Gardiner to essentially manage the affairs of Saskatchewan from his position in the House of Commons in Ottawa. When Douglas scoffed at that idea, the fight was on.

- Tommy Douglas agreed to let his name stand for president of the Saskatchewan CCF Party. In July 1942, with Saskatchewan party leader George Williams still serving overseas, Douglas won the leadership of the Party.
- As 1944 dawned, Tommy Douglas resigned his position as Member of Parliament in Ottawa and returned to Saskatchewan, letting his name stand in the Weyburn riding.
- What nobody saw coming in the 1944 election was a Liberal trouncing. The CCF took 47 of the 52 seats in the Legislature along with 53% per cent of the popular vote. Tommy Douglas, age 39, was now Tommy Douglas MLA and Premier of Saskatchewan.

13

Hard Work and Lots of It

THE TEAM

Premier Douglas set a torrid pace for his Cabinet. He appointed lawyer and former Moose Jaw Mayor John Wesley Corman as Attorney General. Corman's key role was to deal with federal-provincial relations. Woodrow Lloyd, teacher and labour union supporter, was appointed to the Education portfolio and tasked with consolidating the many small school divisions into larger, more cost-effective ones. John Brocklebank from Tisdale was assigned the Municipal Affairs portfolio. Rosetown MLA Jack Douglas was tasked with the Highways and Public Works case file and would soon come to play a role in setting up a Crown Corporation called the Saskatchewan Transportation Company. Former teacher and now MLA for Saskatoon, John Sturdy, was appointed Minister for Reconstruction and Rehabilitation and given a mandate to work with federal Minister of Munitions and Supply, C.D. Howe, to purchase all leftover war materials in Saskatchewan. He worked a deal with Howe whereby Saskatchewan would buy war materials at 6-8% of their assessed value. Sturdy then sold these assets to rural municipalities, school boards, and hospitals at 10% of assessed value. This program saw small towns receiving $25,000 fire engines for only $2,500. Airforce hangars and storage buildings were sold to small towns who repurposed them into curling rinks and skating rinks.

Although overjoyed at being elected, Douglas knew the road ahead would be a rough one. The province's finances were precarious thanks to the preceding ten years of drought and depression. Former Regina alderman and CCF Party veteran Clarence Fines was assigned the dual portfolio of Minister of Public Service and Treasurer. It would fall to Fines to control expenditures, pay interest on the accumulated debt, develop the economy, and find the money to fund new social programs. Fines was also made Deputy Premier. In other words, Fines was tasked with managing practically everything so that Douglas could focus on policy changes to healthcare.

Committed to healthcare reform, Douglas appointed himself Minister of Public Health and took full control of advancing healthcare issues. His election promise to the people had been that money would never be a barrier to people seeking essential care. As Minister, he apprised everyone on social assistance that they would receive free hospital, diagnostic, and doctor services. He made the treatment for cancer and tuberculosis free for all Saskatchewan residents. He hired Johns Hopkins University professor Henry Ernest Sigerist to complete a full review of the provincial health system using a staff of dedicated officials hired from across Canada and the United States.

Of all the MLAs assigned to Cabinet positions, the one that stands out for his aggressive behavior in carrying out his mandate is Joe Phelps. In 1944, Douglas chose Phelps to head up the Ministry of Natural Resources. Phelps had been born in 1899 in Belleville, Ontario. In 1908, he came west with his family who took up homesteading near Wilkie, Saskatchewan. In 1918, he became a district director for the Saskatchewan Grain Growers

Association. In 1928, he became involved with the United Farmers of Canada and then the Farmer-Labour party. This trajectory brought him into contact with Major Coldwell and then into CCF politics.

Phelps was tasked with figuring out the best ways of developing Saskatchewan's rich abundance of natural resources, including oil, natural gas, potash, and uranium, while managing the forests and fish stocks of the north. In his hasty enthusiasm, Phelps made some quick-timed, arguably ill-advised investments in small manufacturing enterprises that ultimately lost money: a shoe factory in Regina, a leather tannery in Regina, a woollen mill in Moose Jaw, a box factory in Prince Albert, and a brick factory in Estevan. So driven to create new entities was Joe Phelps that he earned the nickname "a steam engine wearing pants."

A CYCLONE TEST

The young government was soon taken to task by Nature. On August 15, 1944, a cyclone hit the village of Kamsack, Saskatchewan. The Douglas team moved quickly: the Army was brought in, relief kitchens were set up, Tommy Douglas took to the radio to solicit monetary donations, and the federal government was convinced to provide surplus wartime building materials from its inventory. Kamsack was rebuilt in record time. The Douglas government had met and passed its first test.

A RAPID PACE

In rapid-fire order, the Douglas CCF government passed 76 bills that dealt with issues ranging from farm debt to trade-union rights. Each bill made a change that Douglas had promised during the campaign. He was sharply aware that building the economy required diversification beyond just agriculture. A province focused on wheat alone would find itself in a perilous place if the world price of wheat was to fall.

He is reported to have been cautioned that he was pushing his Cabinet too hard, and introducing change too quickly for the people of Saskatchewan. However, his time in Ottawa arguing against the King Liberals, had taught him the perils of a government that moved too slow.

On one hand, Douglas was pleased with the torrid pace of legislative progress his new government had made. But, on the other hand he realized that Natural Resources Minister Joe Phelps was perhaps moving too fast. The risk was that Phelps and his manufacturing enterprises might be generating the type of publicity that would come to pose a threat to the reputation of the new government.

A Better Civil Service

Douglas also realized that if he was going to move the province forward, he would need a powerful, engaged civil service with greater administrative capacity than the one he inherited. He invited interested men and women from Saskatchewan as well as from across Canada to join the civil service of his new government. Partisan politics would not enter the equation; education and capability would be the key metrics for hire.

One hire of note was a Japanese Canadian, Thomas Shoyama, who made the move from Victoria to Regina to work as a CCF research economist. Another notable hire was Albert Johnson, who had just received his Ph.D from Harvard University. Johnson would one day become the President of the CBC. Today the Johnson Shoyama Business School at the University of Saskatchewan bears their names. Another hire was Weyburn resident Thomas Hector McLeod who had gone to Harvard to obtain a Ph.D in Economics. Later in his career, McLeod would go on to provide service to the Canadian Development Agency.

To better control resource development, Premier Douglas created a cabinet committee called the Economic Advisory and Planning Board. It was chaired by George Woodall Cadbury, a British socialist, whom Douglas had hired in 1945. Cadbury hailed from Birmingham, England.

His grandfather had founded the famous Cadbury chocolate company. While studying economics at Cambridge University, Cadbury's supervisor was none other than the rising star of economics, John Maynard Keynes. As practically any Economics 101 textbook will tell you, Keynes was an advocate for government involvement in an economy facing difficulty. After Cambridge, Cadbury studied economics at the graduate level at the Wharton School of Business at the University of Pennsylvania. During the war, he returned to the UK where he took on the role of Director of Production at the Ministry of Aircraft Production. Cadbury's connections included David Lewis (who would one day be the federal NDP leader). Lewis suggested that Cadbury pay a visit to Saskatchewan to see Premier Douglas. The visit proved fruitful for all concerned. Premier Douglas offered Cadbury the job of setting up and leading the Economic Advisory and Planning Board. Cadbury also was instrumental in creating the Budget Bureau and the Government Finance Office, which today is known as Crown Investments Corporation, the overseer of the various provincial Crown Corporations in Saskatchewan. Under leadership and oversight from the Economic Advisory and Planning Board, the actions of Joe Phelps were slowed to a more reasonable pace.

The Economic Advisory and Planning Board encouraged the creation of fur and fish-marketing cooperatives in northern Saskatchewan so that Cree, Dene, and Métis residents could take greater control of their economic futures. These efforts were met with mixed feelings. Was it the role of government to define the economic future of Indigenous people? Or, was this too colonial in its thinking? Despite the mixed feelings, these cooperative ideas were soon rolled into the Fur Marketing Service and the Fish Board. Crown entities were also set up to provide a market for the vast stands of timber in the north. An air service was created to serve northern communities and to provide air ambulance service. In the central and southern part of the province, the Advisory Board put its stamp of approval on a brick plant, an insurance company, a bus transportation company, and sodium sulphate mining.

FARM SECURITY

In 1944, Saskatchewan saw 185 farm foreclosures. 1945 was looking to be even more dire. The Douglas government passed the *Farm Security Act* which protected the home quarter from foreclosure, and suspended mortgage principal and interest payments in bad years. A bad year was defined as one in which a farmer earned less than $6 per acre of land seeded. This bill created a furor. Both the Supreme Court and the British Privy Council labelled it ultra vires. In other words, Saskatchewan was out of its league. It had no right to dictate to bankers. But Douglas refused to back down. His government next passed a modified version of the Act called the *Exemptions Act*. This piece of legislation further snubbed the banks and stipulated a farmer could keep enough grain to ensure he could seed next year's crop. He could also retain enough machinery and equipment to work the land. The King government in Ottawa was not pleased and decided to push back. It would not be King personally who would do the pushing back. That distinction fell to former Saskatchewan Premier, and now federal Agriculture Minister, Jimmy Gardiner.

JIMMY GARDINER FIGHTS DIRTY

The 1937 crop year had been a disaster. Many farmers harvested scarcely more than three bushels to the acre. When a shortage of seed loomed on the horizon for the 1938 crop year, the Federal government stepped in with cash advances of $16 million to help Saskatchewan farmers buy seed. The one caveat of the loan was that the Saskatchewan government had to guarantee the $16 million. Had a Liberal government been elected in the 1944 Saskatchewan election, it is likely that Ottawa would have written off the $16 million loan. But the Liberals were out. The CCF was in. And now Jimmy Gardiner was tasked with pushing back against Douglas and his *Farm Security* and *Exemptions Act*. The feud was on. It was payback time. Gardiner's opening gambit was to submit an invoice to the province of Saskatchewan for $16 million.

The *Journals of the Legislative Assembly of the Province of Saskatchewan* detail the proceedings in the Legislature during the sitting of early 1945. The facts and figures contained in the proceedings clearly show that Ottawa had extended $16.14 million in seed subsidies. The 1943 revenues for the province including federal subsidies were $27.25 million; government expenses were $26.72 million. The 1944 revenues for the province including federal subsidies were $34.27 million and expenses were $29.79 million. There was not a lot of wiggle room. The province would be hard pressed to deliver on Jimmy Gardiner's demands for a return of $16 million in a timely fashion. Premier Douglas took the entire matter to an arbitration panel, but lost. There was nowhere to turn. The province was now on the hook to repay the federal government. Acrimonious negotiations followed in which the province offered to repay Ottawa at the rate of $400,000 per year for 20 years. Jimmy Gardiner took a hard stance and asked for $1.7 million annually for 10 years (interest included).

SETTLEMENT

As the negotiations were underway to reach a solution, the federal government, in a move to demonstrate how serious it was, withheld $2,272,064 in transfer subsidies to Saskatchewan. To thoroughly drive the point home, Prime Minister King further threatened to disallow the recently passed *Farm Security Act*. Prime Minister King reminded Premier Douglas that Ottawa had the right to do so as per Section 90 of the 1867 *Constitution Act*. This sobering bit of politics propelled both sides to arrive at an agreement in which Saskatchewan would pay $14,196,000 back to Ottawa. Of this, $6,626,000 would be paid in full by July 1948. The remaining balance of $7,570,000 would be paid in annual installment of $700,000 a year extending out to 1956.

The *Journals of the Legislative Assembly of the Province of Saskatchewan* publication for 1945 shows that for the fiscal period March 1945 through March 1946 the projected provincial revenues would be $34.1 million. The projected expenditures (including debt repayment provisions) would be $31.9 million. Things would still be tight, but Saskatchewan would pull through.

To reinforce the message, Clarence Fines and Premier Douglas traveled east to meet with anxious bankers who had purchased Saskatchewan government bonds. In 1944, the 5% bonds due in 1958 were trading at 91 cents on the dollar; enough to make any banker raise his eyebrows. In 1944, the 4% bonds due in 1955 were trading at 84 cents on the dollar; enough to cause a banker some sleepless nights. Once the message was delivered that Saskatchewan was going to survive economically thanks to a reasonable settlement with Ottawa, the 1955 bonds were soon trading at 103 cents on the dollar and the 1958 bonds were soon trading at 113 cents on the dollar. The bankers took a sigh of relief.

HOSPITAL INSURANCE

On January 1, 1947, Premier Douglas (who was also functioning as the Minister of Health) established universal hospital coverage by way of the *Saskatchewan Hospital Insurance Act*. This was the first government-run, single-payer scheme in North America. This Act ensured that residents of Saskatchewan would not be saddled with huge bills for hospital stays. All an individual would have to pay would be a compulsory annual premium of $5 (or up to $30 per family). By the end of 1947, 93% of the population was covered by hospital insurance. Provincial sales tax paid for 20% of the costs, provincial tax levies paid for 20%, and resource royalties were used to pay the remaining 60% of costs.

SOCIAL POLICY

The Douglas team went on to play a leadership role in creating the Saskatchewan Arts Council, the University of Regina, the College of Medicine at the University of Saskatchewan, and an agriculture research station at the University of Saskatchewan. Using surplus war assets, the government made sure small towns and villages had arenas constructed.

School textbooks were provided free of charge to school children. Beer parlors were opened to both sexes. Dining rooms were granted the ability to serve alcohol (except on Sundays). Commenting on the alcohol issue, the Premier is reported to have said: "I would prefer that people not drink at all. But I recognize in a free society that I have no more right to prevent another man drinking than he has the right to force me to drink."

By mid-1946, the government had passed or amended 192 bills. Much of this legislation — focused on changes to human rights, labour law, social security, and education — was the first of its kind anywhere in North America.

People were talking. Was the CCF government moving too fast? It was time to find out. It was time to ask the people.

1948: A FRESH MANDATE

The people delivered their verdict in the June 24, 1948 provincial election. The CCF Party retained its majority, but lost 16 seats including the one held by Joe Phelps. The message for the government to ease up on its pace was received. Commenting on the loss of seats, Premier Douglas mildly chastised the electorate when he referred to the efforts that his government had extended by saying, "Only a small minority might have their toes stepped on, but they tend to remember. The many that have been helped tend to forget." In other words, we passed significant amounts of legislation, but yet you return us to office with fewer seats that before.

With a new mandate from voters, Premier Douglas shifted his focus from social policy to economic policy. Cabinet minister J. H. Brockelbank was moved from the Municipal Affairs portfolio to Natural Resources. He was tasked with identifying and mapping areas of the province where resources were likely to be found and encouraging the private sector to undertake the risks of prospecting and developing the resources. The government plan was to use exploration fees and mining royalties to fund economic policy. Focus also turned to expanding rural electrification, natural gas distribution, and highway development.

Painfully aware of the track record of some of the Crown entities, Premier Douglas made it clear that going forward the goal of the Crown entities that had been created would be threefold:

- To provide good service
- To keep costs for consumer down
- To make a profit (if possible).

This threefold mandate is interesting in its structure. The profitability aspect is listed last along with the words "if possible". This third goal would rear its head in 1957 in the Mossbank debate.

In his capacity as Minister of Health, Premier Douglas pushed for progress in the areas of expanded psychiatric services, creation of mental health clinics, and improved leadership and staff at psychiatric hospitals. Perhaps feeling remorse for his MA thesis on eugenics and perhaps disturbed by his research experience at the Weyburn mental hospital in the 1930s, Premier Douglas wanted to improve the lives of those suffering from mental illness.

POLITICS OF A DIFFERENT SORT

It was now becoming apparent that Tommy Douglas was a different sort of politician. He had a distinct lack of personal vanity. He was interested in the rights of others and believed in setting social, economic, and political goals and working towards them, whether that imperiled his re-election chances or not. Today, politicians are more concerned about gaining office and retaining office. They twist and morph policies, always with an eye on re-election. It would be Premier Douglas' unique lack of focus on just getting re-elected that would guide his decision to debate Ross Thatcher in the not-too-distant future in Mossbank. Will this country ever see another politician whose values parallel those of Tommy Douglas? We can only hope so.

1952: ANOTHER MANDATE

The electorate was pleased with the slow, steady, and efficient governance of the Douglas government. Budget surpluses and the Saskatchewan Power program of rural electrification also added to the electorate's satisfaction. In the 1952 election, the CCF regained some momentum that had been lost in the 1948 election, taking 42 seats and leaving the Liberals with only 11 seats.

Healthcare, however, remained a top priority for the Premier. He envisioned a program where residents of Saskatchewan would have all medically necessary expenses paid for. But the issue was money. What was really needed was help from Ottawa. Unfortunately, the Liberal government under Louis St. Laurent was not interested in giving the province the money. In fact, Ottawa wanted to ignore the healthcare issue completely.

1956: ANOTHER MAJORITY

The province continued to slowly mark progress through the 1950s. At the 1956 Legislature sitting it was made clear the government was fighting Ottawa for better freight rates for grain farmers. To improve transportation for farmers in the province, a $50 million plan was announced to create a grid system of roads throughout the rural areas. Uranium mining was now well underway in the north. Oil drilling activity was robust and hard rock mineral exploration activity was setting records. A total of three million acres were being intensely drilled and explored for potash. A cement plant, a sewer pipe plant, and a wire & cable plant were being established. As well, a steel plant at the north end of Regina was being built (Interprovincial Pipe and Steel, now owned by Evraz). The program of rural electrification would see a total of 40,000 farms along with all villages and towns electrified by the end of 1956. Telephone service was also being expanded thanks to the installation of a series of microwave frequency relay towers across the province. In addition, the ice had finally broken in Ottawa on the subject of healthcare. The St. Laurent government agreed, at least in principle, to a program of cost sharing for hospital and diagnostic services.

The people of Saskatchewan were generally happy with the progress being made. In June 1956 the CCF Party was returned to office with 36 seats. The Liberals took 14 and the Social Credit Party 3 seats.

The healthcare cost sharing issue would soon take another big step forward. The political turf in Ottawa shifted dramatically in 1957 when Saskatchewan's own John Diefenbaker and his Conservative Party narrowly edged out the Liberals. Mr. Diefenbaker's mother was confined to a hospital bed in Prince Albert, Saskatchewan. Diefenbaker shared Douglas' concerns over healthcare and suggested that he would create a federal-provincial cost sharing program for healthcare that would take effect on July 1, 1958. In the end, Diefenbaker's program failed to launch.

Meanwhile, the events that were shaping Saskatchewan were also having an impact on a politician from Moose Jaw, Saskatchewan – Ross Thatcher.

- The new Premier faced an economy that had just endured a decade of drought and depression. Nevertheless, he set a torrid pace. In short order, the Douglas CCF government passed 76 bills that dealt with issues ranging from farm debt to trade-union rights.
- He also reformed the civil service, reaching out to educated men and women from across Canada to join the civil service of his new government.
- The Economic Advisory and Planning Board was created to kickstart a series of new Crown Corporations to ensure a robust

post-war economy for Saskatchewan. The track record and management of these Crown entities would underpin the 1957 Great Debate in Mossbank.

- In early 1947, Douglas established universal hospital coverage by way of the *Saskatchewan Hospital Insurance Act*. This was the first government-run, single-payer scheme in North America. All an individual would have to pay would be an annual premium of $5 (or up to $30 per family).

- Douglas proved himself a different sort of politician. He had a distinct lack of personal vanity. He believed in setting social, economic, and political goals and working towards them, whether that imperiled his re-election chances or not.

- The CCF was returned to power in the 1948, 1952, and 1956 elections.

- His healthcare initiatives took a big step forward in 1957 when John Diefenbaker's Conservatives defeated the Liberals. Diefenbaker shared Douglas's concerns over healthcare and suggested a federal-provincial cost sharing program for healthcare.

14

From Neville, Saskatchewan, Ross Thatcher Came

Ross Thatcher's father, Wilbert Thatcher, was born in 1888 in Arthur, Ontario near present day Guelph, Ontario.

In 1907, young Wilbert made his way west to Saskatchewan where he found employment as a printer at weekly newspapers; first in the village of Qu'Appelle and later in the village of Caron. He continued to work as a printer until 1912 when he accepted a job as a traveling salesman for the International Harvester Company.

In 1915 he entered the hardware business in the village of Neville, Saskatchewan with business partner Percy Prowse.

In 1917, Wilbert Thatcher was 29 and his wife, Marjorie Belle Price, was 26. Marjorie gave birth to a son, Ross on May 24, 1917. Wilbert and Marjorie would go on to have four more children: Clarke, Edward, Hugh, and Joan.

By 1918, Wilbert Thatcher and Percy Prowse found their business partnership relations strained and decided to go their separate ways. Wilbert is on record as having said of Mr. Prowse, "We were good friends in business and we were good friends in opposition."

Wilbert set up a hardware store in Limerick, Saskatchewan with branches in Lafleche, Melaval, Valor, and Wood Mountain. In 1928, with some financing help from the hardware wholesaler Marshall-Wells Company, he purchased a hardware store in Moose Jaw. This location became the focal point for his hardware empire. Even as the economy slumped into recession after the 1929 stock market crash, Mr. Thatcher maintained his focus on tight inventory control and excellent customer service, even going so far as extending credit to desperate farm families. Young Ross Thatcher grew up in and around hardware, learning these finer points of the business from his dad.

Ross was a sharp student and graduated from high school in Moose Jaw in 1932 at the age of 15. He made his way to Queen's University in Kingston, Ontario where he excelled in studies towards his Economics degree. Following graduation, he was offered a lucrative job as the executive assistant to a Mr. McLean—the Vice President of Canada Packers in Toronto. One of Thatcher's tasks was to prepare a weekly profit and loss statement for his boss. He soon realized that this task was no different than the profit and loss calculations he used to do for his father's hardware business. Control the costs, deliver good service, provide a good product, and Canada Packers would make money. This philosophy would one day come to influence his political viewpoints as well.

While working for Canada Packers, Ross made several trips back to Moose Jaw. On one of these visits, he met Peggie who had been born Adrah Leone McNaughton around 1916 in Worthing, England to Charles and Flora McNaughton. When she was a young child, her family immigrated to Canada and settled in Moose Jaw, where her father owned and operated the Capital Ice Company. At the time Ross and Peggie met, she was writing articles for the women's pages of the Moose *Jaw Times Herald*. She was a volunteer with the Howard Johnson Society, a member of St. Andrew's United Church, a supporter of the Girl Guides, and a member of the Saskatchewan Liberal Women's Association. She was also a locally renowned badminton player.

Ross Thatcher and Peggie McNaughton were married in January of 1938. They had one son, Colin, born on August 25, 1938 in Toronto, Ontario. Shortly afterwards, in 1939, Wilbert Thatcher fell ill and summoned son Ross to come home from Toronto to take over the hardware business. He further showed his entrepreneurial mettle when he used his savings from his Canada Packers job to secure financing on 10 rental houses in Moose Jaw reasoning that should war break out, there would be a demand for housing after the war as soldiers returned home. He would eventually be proven correct and would later sell many of the houses at a profit. He parlayed the profits into the purchase of a cattle ranch at Caron, Saskatchewan near Moose Jaw.

War on the European front was looming. William Lyon Mackenzie King was Prime Minister. He was wary of seeing Canada plow head first into a war. A powerful orator in the House of Commons, Douglas was hammering on the King government for not having done enough to help the Saskatchewan farmer who has just endured the peak of a drought and insect infestation. Meanwhile in Regina, Saskatchewan Liberal Premier, William Patterson, was refusing to run a deficit to help the province through the tough economic times. No doubt, the plight of the Saskatchewan farmer was having a negative impact on the hardware business.

In Moose Jaw, Ross Thatcher began to voice displeasure with Saskatchewan politics. No doubt, having worked for a major corporation in a major Canadian city had helped to shape his views. Thatcher felt that the Saskatchewan economy could do better and that the government had to step up to the plate and play a bigger role. His beliefs soon led him to join the CCF Party.

In 1942, he was elected to Moose Jaw council for a two-year term. This whetted his appetite for elected office. What was not known at the time was that Ross Thatcher would one day go on to be Premier of Saskatchewan. This journey would see his career trajectory intersect with that of Tommy Douglas.

- Ross Thatcher was born in Neville, Saskatchewan on May 24, 1917.
- He was a sharp student and graduated from high school in Moose Jaw in 1932 at the age of 15. After graduating from Queen's University with a degree in Economics, he was offered a lucrative job as the executive assistant to the Vice President of Canada Packers in Toronto. He learned that the strategy for making a profit was to control costs, deliver a good service, and provide a good product. This philosophy would one day come to influence his political viewpoints as well.
- In 1939, when his father took ill, Thatcher came home from Toronto to take over his father's hardware business in Moose Jaw.
- Ross Thatcher soon began to voice displeasure with Saskatchewan politics. He felt the Saskatchewan economy could do better and that the government had to step up to the plate and play a bigger role. His beliefs soon led him to join the CCF Party.

15

The End of the
War Nears

War at any time in history is a huge economic dislocation. During World
War II, manufacturing efforts in Canada shifted to making supplies and
munitions for the combat effort. Government funds footed the bill.
One of the consequences of this economic dislocation was a shortage of
consumer goods.

As the possibility of German surrender became a distinct possibility,
private enterprise started feeling uncertain. An end to the war in Europe
would mean the production of supplies and munitions would soon no
longer be needed. But what would the state of the economy be? What
consumer goods should now be made? Would the soldiers coming home
be able to find jobs? To what extent would government step in to help the
post-war economy? The dislocated economy was posing more questions
than answers.

Government economists would have looked back at the aftermath of
World War I for guidance. That post-war period was one of turmoil that

quickly saw the North American economy fall backwards into recession as demand for war supplies and munitions faded. Soldiers returning home found a bleak employment situation. Germany, meanwhile, could not afford to import goods from North America because the German government was being forced to make sizeable financial reparations for the damage done in Europe. Would the same scenario play out this time?

LIBERAL RECONSTRUCTION COUNCIL

In February, 1944, the Liberal government of William Patterson was aware that the end of the war was becoming likely. Patterson was also aware that Saskatchewan needed to get its economy firing on all cylinders. He took steps to create a Reconstruction Council. Details on what this Council proposed are sparse. The Opposition CCF Party used the creation of the Reconstruction Council to express its strategies for the Saskatchewan economy.

At the early 1944 Legislative sitting. CCF MLAs Brocklebank and Johnston laid out a seven step platform they thought the governing Liberals should embrace:

(1)   Flax crushing;
(2)   Tanning and processing of hides;
(3)   Woollen Mill;
(4)   Canning and processing of vegetables;
(5)   Building material industries for the production of clay products, lumber, pulp wood products and glass;
(6)   Manufacture of farm machinery and builders' hardware from scrap iron; and
(7)   Taking action where projects are found to be economical.

CCF Party MLA Joe Phelps also weighed in with his wish list of nine items he thought the Liberals should aim for,

(1) "Development of new power sites and acquisition of main existing ones in order to provide mass production of power on a province-wide network of electrical energy to all main points, with due regard for future industrial expansion within Saskatchewan; further development of our great resources of the north; and a plentiful supply to our most thickly populated rural areas, together with other parts adjacent to lines constructed in order to make possible mass consumption at the lowest cost.

(2) Increased exploratory and survey work to determine the value of undeveloped resources in Saskatchewan with a view to their social development.

(3) A programme of conservation of all our resources and redrafting of timber regulations.

(4) Processing of a much larger percentage of coal production in order to improve the heat value and derive greater use of its by-products.

(5) The introduction of a tax on all natural resources now being developed on all properties where the mineral rights have not been reserved to the Crown.

(6) The establishment of a Provincial Marketing Board with power to take delivery of and market all timber and timber products, coal and other materials produced from our natural resources, thus providing the consumer with finished products at a lower cost.

(7) The establishment of a provincial fur exchange.

(8) Establishment of cold storage facilities at suitable points to ensure preservation of a supply of northern fresh water fish.

(9) The extension of regular air routes to northern points in the province for the purpose of passenger traffic, aerial patrol and transportation of supplies into these northern points".

Despite the creation of the Reconstruction Council, time was running out for the Patterson government. The last election had been in 1938. What normally would have been an election in 1942-43 was delayed because of the war. With the end of the war now a real possibility, Patterson decided to ask the people of Saskatchewan for a new mandate.

Unfortunately, for Mr. Patterson and his Liberals, they were soundly denied the opportunity to remain in office. The people of Saskatchewan opted for a new political direction with the CCF Party winning 47 of 52 seats. The question to ponder is, had T.C. Douglas and the CCF Party not come into power in the June 1944 election, would Patterson's Liberals have taken some of these CCF ideas and put them into play? If so, what would this have meant for the Saskatchewan economy?

- Aware that the war would soon end, government economists no doubt would have looked to the aftermath of World War I for guidance. That post-war period saw the North American economy fall into recession as demand for war supplies and munitions faded. Soldiers returning home found a bleak employment situation. Germany, saddled by reparation payment obligations could not afford to import goods from North America. Would the same scenario play out this time?
- The Patterson Liberal government was also aware that Saskatchewan needed to get its economy firing on all cylinders and moved to create a Reconstruction Council.
- Details on what this Council proposed were sparse. Instead of just criticizing the Reconstruction Council, the Opposition CCF Party created a platform that expressed its strategies for the Saskatchewan economy.

16

The CCF Approach to
the Post-war Economy

The manufacturing sector in western Canada suffered in the aftermath of the economic dislocation caused by WW I. Douglas and his CCF party concluded that the WW II economic dislocation would be different. They felt that the manufacturing sector would benefit this time around. The Douglas government decided to take proactive action in the form of Crown Corporations that would kickstart the Saskatchewan economy which was primarily agriculture based.

What the Douglas government did not factor into their reasoning was the role the US government would play in the World War II economic dislocation. The relatively unscathed United States quickly emerged as the de-facto world power. Thanks to the *Bretton Woods Conference*, the US Dollar would become the global reserve currency. The *World Bank* would be created. The *Marshall Plan* laid down by President Truman through his *Economic Recovery Act* would see money spent in a big way to rebuild Europe. The *Allied Council* under the leadership of General Douglas MacArthur would take bold steps to rebuild Japan. While private enterprise after World War I was paralyzed, there would be no uncertainty this time. As the Douglas government made moves to establish Crown Corporations, more efficient private sector manufacturers rose to the challenge across North America. The relatively inefficient government Crown structures in Saskatchewan would eventually find themselves facing stiff competition.

The premise behind the Crown corporation model was summed up by Douglas, "It is my intention, first, to use the available revenue of this province to expand our social services; second, to eliminate inequities and injustices from our taxation system; third, to find new sources of revenue wherever they can be found without increasing the burden of the common people of this province; and, finally, to utilize all available investment capital for the development of Saskatchewan's resources. In short, the financial policy of this Government, like every other policy, is designed to serve the people. This is the basic principle of the CCF; it is the basic principle of this government."

He further stated, "It is the feeling of my government that the day is past when it can be left to the forces of private enterprise exclusively to develop the resources of the community and to organize its business activity. The modern economy is a complex one that demands control and direction if disaster and chaos are to be averted. Well aware of the obstacles confronting any attempt at planning on a provincial scale, my government remains of the opinion that much can be done to plan in such a manner that the economic activities of the people of this Province may be carried on more efficiently."

Just as the private manufacturing sector across North America was poised to gain momentum, Douglas was expressing his viewpoint that the forces of private enterprise could not be relied upon. This political viewpoint would have negative consequences that would eventually form the basis for the Mossbank 1957 debate.

Legislature proceedings along with annual financial statements from various Saskatchewan Crown entities reveal that a three-pronged approach was taken in forming the various Crown Corporations: provide very good service, provide said service at favorable prices, and make a profit (if possible). This third prong would be the problem child.

The Douglas government could easily have started providing new services and consumer products within the structure of a government ministry or department. But this would have left the Minister in charge. By establishing a Crown entity, a corporation was created within the overall government structure. The corporation would be overseen by a member of the Douglas bureaucracy; the bureaucracy of highly educated people he had hand-picked.

The Douglas government then began to apply pressure to the federal government for economic assistance. The following verbiage from the March 1945 Legislative sitting shows the list of demands made on Ottawa:

That this Assembly, realizing that the agricultural industry of Canada must be placed on a permanently sound economic basis if the predominantly agricultural provinces are to achieve and maintain their full and proper status in Confederation, urges upon the Government of Canada the necessity of establishing, to this end:

(1) *Floor prices on all staple farm products as the most effective method of maintaining maximum farm production and stabilizing the agricultural industry; but that such floor prices should provide to agricultural producers their proper share of the national income; and such floor prices should be guaranteed at all times for at least two years in advance for cereal grains, and for at least five years in advance for livestock, poultry and their products;*

(2) *Legislation to protect the farmer's equity in his land, home and machinery;*

(3)   *Assistance to returned men and others who wish to farm co-operatively;*

(4)   *Public ownership of plants manufacturing farm implements and supplies and, where expansion of the industry is necessary, the conversion of Government-owned war plants for the purpose;*

(5)   *Assistance to co-operatives for the distribution of farm machinery and supplies;*

(6)   *Co-operative or public ownership of the major processing and wholesale distributing facilities for farm products;*

(7)   *Adequate storage and refrigeration facilities and the application of the "ever normal granary" principle to major staples;*

(8)   *Means for extensive development of the industrial utilization of farm products;*

(9)   *A comprehensive national crop insurance scheme to be applied on an individual basis at premiums no greater than the minimum cost of service;*

(10) *Farm credit at the cost of service;*

(11) *Marketing Boards, representative of producer and consumer, for the orderly grading and marketing of all farm products;*

(12) *The present Wheat Board as a Grain Board with adequate producer and consumer representation to handle all grain; providing initial payments and participation certificates; the initial payment for wheat for the crop year 1945 to be not less than $1.25 per bushel, and the initial payment for coarse grains to be not less than the present ceiling prices for coarse grains, plus the equalization payments now being paid;*

(13) *Export and Import Boards for the regulation and encouragement of Canada's foreign trade in agricultural as well as other commodities;*

(14) *That the price of cheese for 1945 be set at 25 cents a pound, factory shipping point, plus the quality premium now paid; and that the subsidy on butterfat be fixed at 13 cents per pound until October 1st, 1945 and at 15 cents from that date to May 1st, 1946. And, further, that fluid milk subsidies be continued at 55 cents per*

> *hundred pounds throughout the year, and that in any health plan*
> *for Canada the place of fluid milk should be featured;*
>
> (15) *A Board of Livestock Commissioners with producer representation,*
> *and having similar p*owers to those of the Board of Grain
> Commissioners;

When it became apparent that Ottawa could not be counted on to help, Premier Douglas and his CCF government decided to forge ahead by themselves and sold $5 million of 10-Year bonds (bearing a coupon of 3% interest) to residents of Saskatchewan. The process of creating Crown Corporations then got underway in earnest.

The Opposition aggressively targeted the activities and decisions of the Douglas government. At the 1947 sitting, Premier Douglas, under pressure from the Opposition, sought to set straight the issue of accounting for the Crown entities. He said, "The criticism has been raised that the Crown Corporations do not pay interest on advances from the Treasury. But the people of Saskatchewan, through their government, are in actuality the shareholders, rather than the creditors, of the Corporations. As a consequence, they will receive dividends from their investment, as the Corporations earn profits to be paid into the funds of the government. These dividends, indeed, may amount to much more than normal interest on advances. Nor are the Crown Corporations merely money-making operations designed to earn profits. They serve, as well, a distinct social purpose and their policies are guided always with regard to social considerations."

This description of how the Crown entities should function is attractive indeed. But, as the Opposition would point out repeatedly in the years to come, many of these Crowns were not making money; they were consuming money.

- The Douglas government appreciated that the Saskatchewan economy was agriculture-based, not manufacturing-based and they decided to take action engage to develop the production of manufactured goods in an effort to broaden the Saskatchewan economy away from its agrarian focus.

- What the Douglas government did not factor in to their reasoning was that the relatively unscathed United States was now the de-facto world power. The US Dollar would become the global reserve currency. The *World Bank*, the *Marshall Plan*, and the *Truman Economic Recovery Act* would see money spent in a big way to get Europe rebuilt quickly. The Allied Council under the leadership of General Douglas MacArthur would take similar bold steps to rebuild Japan.

- Private sector industry across North America rose to the challenge. As the Douglas government made moves to establish Crown Corporations, more efficient private sector manufacturers rose to the challenge.

17

Ross Thatcher
Goes to Ottawa

THE 1945 FEDERAL ELECTION

Prime Minister King reminded people that the war was now over and it was time to build a new social order. He promised:

- $750 million to provide land, jobs and business support for veterans
- $400 million of public spending to build housing
- $250 million for a family allowance program
- the creation of an Industrial Development Bank
- loans to farmers, and floor prices for agricultural products
- tax reductions.

Although his promises were big and bold, what plagued King during the 1945 campaign was the lingering controversy over wartime conscription and the *National Resources Mobilization Act* (NRMA). Participation in the war was a delicate political issue. Those who had volunteered felt that it was unfair that others their same age had opted to sit at home while the war dragged on in Europe. English Canada was strongly in favour of conscripting more men into the war effort. The Duplessis government in Quebec, however, made it very clear that Quebec was opposed to conscripting men into service. To gain favour with the Quebec electorate, King tried to hold off on conscripting men into the fight, but by 1944 he could hold off no longer. Of the 13,000 conscripted men that left Canada headed for the war, only 2,463 saw action in the field before the war ended. However, of these, 69 lost their lives. The King government would pay a heavy price at the polls as a result of this contentious conscription policy decision.

When the votes were counted, 18 of 21 federal ridings in Saskatchewan had gone to the CCF Nationally, King's Liberal Party took 118 seats (a loss of 61 seats), the Conservatives 66 seats (a gain of 28), the CCF 28 seats (a gain of 20) and the Social Credit Party 13 seats (a gain of 3). King lost his bid for re-election in the Prince Albert riding to the CCF candidate.

Ross Thatcher's experience on Moose Jaw council made him hungry for a deeper involvement in politics. In 1945, he ran in the federal election in the Moose Jaw riding as the CCF Party candidate. He steam-rolled to victory, taking 9,831 votes. Liberal incumbent John Ross only garnered 5,862 votes.

Ross Thatcher with his degree in Economics, his hardware business experience, and his experience at a major Canadian corporation was a man on a mission. He wanted change and he wanted it now.

1949 FEDERAL ELECTION

In the aftermath of his defeat, Prime Minister King quickly orchestrated a by-election in a safe riding in Ontario to regain his seat in the Commons. Although he won the by-election, he was worn out. During his political career, he had been elected to the House of Commons sixteen times. His various electoral wins had come from ridings in three provinces, making him the most diverse politician in Canadian history to that point. In 1948, he decided to retire after a 32-year-long career. The Liberal Party elected Quebec MP Louis St. Laurent to lead the party. St. Laurent's slogan was "You Never Had It So Good." With that slogan in hand, St. Laurent called an election and asked the electorate for a fresh mandate. After the votes were counted, the Liberals were returned to power with 191 seats (a gain of 73 seats from 1945), the largest majority in Canadian politics to that point in time. The Conservatives under George Drew took 41 seats, a loss of 24 seats from the previous election. One of the Conservative MPs returning to Ottawa was Saskatchewan's John Diefenbaker from the Lake Centre riding. The CCF Party under Major Coldwell took 13 seats, a loss of 15 seats from the previous election. Of the 13 seats won, only 5 were in Saskatchewan; quite a departure from the 18 seats won in the 1945 election.

AT ODDS

Ross Thatcher soon found himself at odds with CCF Party. He personally felt that if private sector capital was not willing to invest, then government should step up and take a leadership role. He came to feel that the CCF saw the private sector as a dominant class that sought to control the means of production and the distribution of wealth in an economy. He concluded that the CCF Party was misguided.

Initially, the Party tolerated him as a maverick. This label was supported by the fact that he seldom socialized with other Party members. The re-arming of post-war Germany further emboldened his maverick status; the CCF party was of the opinion that Germany should be allowed to re-arm itself of its own accord but Thatcher felt any re-arming should be done under the scrutiny of NATO. He broke ranks on the subsequent vote in the House of Commons.

In an effort to reel him in, Coldwell and the Party brass ordered him to support the CCF position in the coming budgetary debate. He was further told never to stray from the Party line again. In the budget debate, the CCF wanted the Liberal government to impose higher corporate taxes. Thatcher felt that this policy position was being driven by the Party affiliation with the big Ontario labour unions. He felt the CCF was losing touch with the western farmer. Moreover, the CCF wanted the government to provide more social benefits, regardless of the cost. This did not sit well with Thatcher at all.

1953 FEDERAL ELECTION

The 1953 federal election saw an improvement for Major Coldwell and his CCF Party. Louis St. Laurent and his Liberals scored another majority, taking 169 seats; a drop of 22 from the last election. The Conservatives took 51 seats, a gain of 10 from the last election. Once again, Saskatchewan's John Diefenbaker was re-elected. The CCF took 23 seats, a gain of 10 from the last election. Of the 23 seats won, 11 were in Saskatchewan; an improvement of six from the last election. In Moose Jaw, Ross Thatcher waltzed to victory with 12,436 votes. His nearest rival, James Gemmell managed only 6,021 votes.

Despite this recent improvement in seat numbers, the CCF Party had not made significant progress in seat numbers since the 1945 election. At issue was a theme that was finding its way into mainstream vocabulary: *Communism.* Supporters of the CCF Party in the early 1950s were being equated with Communism and the Soviet Union. The driving force behind this unrealistic and unfounded insinuation was groups who supported the Conservative Party.

To counter this ridiculous rhetoric, the CCF Party began working to reposition itself. At the 1956 Party convention, a policy platform was adopted which was labeled the *Winnipeg Declaration.* This platform was designed to replace the 1933 *Regina Manifesto.* This new policy position stated that the Party would aim for a centrist political stance that involved public, private, and co-operative enterprises all working together in the people's interest. But the platform also made clear that economic expansion accompanied by widespread suffering and injustice would not be deemed to be desirable social progress.

Leading up to its 1956 release, MP Ross Thatcher would have had a close-up view of the new platform. With his entrepreneurial background, Queen's University education, and corporate insights, he grew disappointed with Major Coldwell and the direction of the Party.

Unable to influence Coldwell's thinking, Ross Thatcher broke ranks with the CCF Party and announced his decision to sit as an Independent MP for his Moose Jaw riding. It was not long before Prime Minister St. Laurent asked Thatcher to run as a Liberal in the next election.

Around the time that Thatcher made his decision to leave the CCF Party, the St. Laurent Liberal government was under fire from the Conservative opposition for what the Conservatives deemed to be overspending under The *Defense Production Act.* The early 1950s were a time of concern over the growing threat of Communism. In 1951, the Department of Defense Production had been created and given sole authority to procure supplies for the Department of National Defense. In the event of another global conflict, Canada would be ready to participate.

At the time, 50 cents of every tax dollar was being spent on defense procurement; everything from bootlaces to bullets. In 1952, Chief Auditor George Currie, assigned to examine the Department of National Defense, uncovered a tangled mess of corruption. Hundreds of millions of dollars had been paid to un-named contractors. An order for 29,630 teapots had been made at a time when military mess halls did not even use teapots. Nearly two million neckties were ordered; enough to last for many years. One of the big-ticket items George Currie found was the cumulative expenditure of $121 million on the Avro Arrow jet project. The list of excess expenditures went on and on. The Conservatives demanded a Royal Commission to get to the bottom of the corruption.

The mid-1950s were also a time of vociferous energy policy debate. The St. Laurent government wanted a natural gas pipeline to move western natural gas to eastern markets. St. Laurent's minister of Trade and Commerce, C. D. Howe, assembled a consortium of Canadian and American investors to fund the Trans Canada Pipeline project. The CCF Party argued that the pipeline should be wholly government owned. The Conservatives argued that there should be no American investors allowed to participate. Between early May and early June 1956, debate raged in the Commons. Time was running out. Sections of pipe had already been fabricated and if any pipe-laying progress was to be realized in 1956, construction had to start soon. Late one evening at an extended sitting of the House to debate the pipeline issue, Liberal convert Ross Thatcher rose to his feet in the House of Commons. He knew an election writ could be dropped at any time. He knew he would be facing the Saskatchewan electorate on a Liberal ticket. He had to start drawing attention to himself. During his late evening speech, he voiced his opposition to the CCF calls for government ownership of the Trans Canada pipeline—but in a clever way. His carefully crafted comments not only supported the Liberal position on the pipeline, but they took an aim at Saskatchewan Premier Tommy Douglas and the overall concept of government ownership. Thatcher was hitting two birds with one stone, so to speak. According to the House of Commons' Hansard, Thatcher said: "I say tonight that the Saskatchewan program of socialization was born in high hopes and with laudable aspirations. But today it is apparent that the program has been bogged down in a morass of bungling, red tape, inefficiency, and inexperience. I say there is not a single Saskatchewan Crown Corporation that has operated in the black for a reasonable length of time without special privileges or compulsion of some kind. I say the program has been a tragedy and a very costly fiasco. I think it has been a dismal failure. At one time I believed in public ownership, but after holding office for 14 years, I am now absolutely convinced that public ownership should only be used under special circumstances. Generally speaking, people simply will not work for the government in business as efficiently as they will for private enterprise."

The message was, government ownership of the Trans Canada Pipeline project would not work. To drive home his point, Thatcher went on to cite the recent financial results of the Saskatchewan leather tannery, shoe factory, Housing Corporation, woollen mill, and brick plant. He labeled these to be financial failures that had cost the taxpayers dearly. He argued that any Saskatchewan Crown Corporations that had made money had done so "…because they enjoyed either government compulsion or some kind of monopoly privilege."

This criticism would be repeated a year later in Mossbank, Saskatchewan, and this time directly to Premier Douglas.

To bring the pipeline arguments to an end, the St. Laurent government finally took a bold step and invoked closure of debate. This move would come back to haunt St. Laurent in the 1957 election.

SUEZ CRISIS

St. Laurent's domestic political issues were further complicated when global geopolitical tensions boiled over in 1956. The 120-mile-long Suez Canal had opened in 1869. It had been constructed to connect the Indian Ocean to the Mediterranean Sea by way of the Red Sea. The overarching goal was to provide a shorter shipping route to get oil from the Middle East to Europe. The canal was jointly operated by a British/French consortium as part the 1936 *Anglo-Egyptian Treaty*. Leading up to 1956, Egypt, under leadership of Gamal Nasser, had developed plans to build a power dam project at Aswan on the Nile River. The US government expressed a willingness to help finance the dam project. In July 1956, the US government reneged on its financing plans. An angry Nasser responded by nationalizing the Suez Canal. He announced a plan to levy tolls on oil-carrying freighters passing through the canal. The money earned from the tolls would pay for the Aswan Dam project. Britain, France, and Israel quickly responded to Nasser's move. In October 1956, troops had advanced to within 40 kilometers of the canal. When Nasser refused to concede, bombing began.

Britain, France, and Israel made their bombing advances without apprising the US and other NATO countries of their plan. This created a furor in Washington and in Moscow. Premier Nikita Khrushchev threatened to rain bombs down on Europe unless Britain, France, and Israel withdrew their troops. President Dwight Eisenhower demanded that all sides back down immediately. In the House of Commons, St. Laurent asked his Foreign Minister Lester Pearson to get involved. Pearson began proposing that a contingent of Peacekeeping troops be sent in to restore order along the Suez. The Conservatives shouted that the St. Laurent and Pearson proposal of Peacekeeping troops was a failure by Canada to support the military actions of Britain. In the end, after intense negotiation, the Peacekeeping solution was adopted and by March of 1957, Nasser re-opened the Canal.

St. Laurent was a battered man. A defense spending scandal. A toxic pipeline debate. Geopolitical tensions. Accusations of a lack of support for Britain.

1957 ELECTION CALL

In late 1956, Conservative leader George Drew fell ill and was forced to step away from politics. At a hotly contested leadership convention, Saskatchewan MP John Diefenbaker prevailed and was named Party leader. He immediately embarked on a cross-Canada tour to condemn the St. Laurent Liberals and to promote the Conservative platform. St. Laurent was squeezed. He needed a fresh mandate. He called a federal election for June 10, 1957.

This was the opportunity Ross Thatcher was waiting for. Time to get re-elected to the House of Commons; this time as a Liberal in the riding of Assiniboia in southern Saskatchewan. The focus for candidate Thatcher would be the Douglas government, its Crown Corporations, and the perils of government ownership.

HAZEN ARGUE

The federal riding of Assiniboia was a big one. It carved out a rectangular pattern; running from the US border to just north of Mossbank and from Weyburn west to Rockglen. Thatcher would have a challenge on his hands. The incumbent MP in the riding was skilled CCF politician Hazen Argue. Hazen Argue has been born in Moose Jaw in January 1921. His parents owned a farm southeast of Moose Jaw near the tiny village of Kayville. When Hazen was five years old, the family rented out their farm and moved to nearby Avonlea, Saskatchewan where his dad started a farm machinery business. Hazen Argue graduated from the University of Saskatchewan in 1944 with a degree in Agriculture. After graduation from university, he wasted little time in turning his attention to politics. In 1945, at the age of 24, he was one of the many CCF candidates elected to the House of Commons. Most certainly he would have become well acquainted with Ross Thatcher. It is thought that Thatcher had opted to run in a rural riding because he perceived there would be better support for the Liberal platform. The one data point Thatcher would have used in his political calculus was from the 1952 election when he eclipsed the Liberal candidate in the Moose Jaw riding by over 6,000 votes. Meantime in the rural Assiniboia riding, MP Argue had surpassed the Liberal candidate by only 3,300 votes.

- In 1945, Ross Thatcher ran in the federal election in the Moose Jaw riding as the CCF candidate. The pivotal issue in the 1945 election was military conscription, a subject that had divided the country. When the votes were counted, 18 of 21 federal ridings in Saskatchewan had gone to the CCF. Ross Thatcher was now headed to The House of Commons in Ottawa.

- Thatcher soon found himself at odds with CCF Party leadership. He felt that if private sector capital was not willing to invest, then government should step up and take a leadership role. His idea was ignored. He began to sense the CCF did not trust the private sector. He concluded that the CCF Party was mis-guided. Ross Thatcher, MP was now becoming Ross Thatcher, maverick.

- In the 1953 election Thatcher again waltzed to victory. The CCF Party then began to reposition itself, aiming for a centrist political stance that involved public, private, and co-operative enterprises all working together in the people's best interest.

- This was not good enough for Ross Thatcher. He broke ranks with the CCF Party and began sitting as an Independent MP.

- Prime Minister St. Laurent soon asked Thatcher to run as a Liberal in the next election. This presented a difficult issue for Thatcher. The Moose Jaw riding was a CCF stronghold. Running on a Liberal ticket there would be futile. He needed another riding. More importantly, he needed some publicity.

- In the House of Commons, he began criticizing how Saskatchewan Premier Tommy Douglas was using Crown Corporations to run the province.

- Thatcher would soon get all the publicity he wanted. In 1956, Saskatchewan MP John Diefenbaker became the federal Conservative Party leader. He immediately began to condemn the St. Laurent Liberals. Prime Minister St. Laurent was squeezed. He needed a fresh mandate. He called a federal election for June 10, 1957.

- This was the opportunity Ross Thatcher was waiting for. Time to get re-elected to the House of Commons; this time as a Liberal in the riding of Assiniboia in southern Saskatchewan. His opponent – incumbent CCF MP, Hazen Argue.

18

Reconstruction and Housing Crowns

SASKATCHEWAN RECONSTRUCTION HOUSING CORPORATION

Veterans returning home from war soon realized that housing was hard to find. The Douglas government started to put pressure on Ottawa to assist with creating additional housing units. Premier Douglas stated, "it is estimated that, at the present time, we need in the Dominion of Canada from 500,000 to 700,000 new houses. We need in the Province of Saskatchewan anywhere from 40,000 to 50,000 new houses. Under the Federal Government's *National Housing Act*, the total number of houses built in this province from the time the Act was passed in 1937 until the end of 1944, was 61. That is a poor makeshift; it is a pretty pathetic contribution to a situation that calls for 40,000 to 50,000 new houses in this province. The federal government says that, in the next year, they hope somewhere between 40,000 and 50,000 will be built in the whole of Canada. That is totally inadequate; it is something like feeding a peanut to an elephant when the requirement is from 500,000 to 700,000 throughout Canada and between 40,000 and 50,000 in Saskatchewan alone."

At the March, 1945, Legislature sitting, the Premier announced, "My government is negotiating with the Crown Assets Allocation Committee to obtain military and air force establishments and equipment for socially useful purposes. Any buildings so obtained during the continuance of the war are to be maintained in such condition that they may be readily reconverted to military uses." The government then proceeded with creating housing units under a Crown structure called the Saskatchewan Reconstruction Housing Corporation. This Crown structure was brought into existence, not by a vote in the Legislature, but with the stroke of a pen using an Order in Council.

In early 1946, Premier Douglas noted, "The Reconstruction Housing Corporation has assisted veterans in securing housing facilities in the present emergency. In spite of the prevailing shortage of materials, some 200 self-contained living units have been provided for returned men's families, and dormitory and messing accommodation for 1,000 men attending the university and vocational training schools."

To the end of 1946, the Corporation had been given $508,500 from provincial coffers and had received grants from Canada Mortgage and Housing (CMHC) in the amount of $133,100. This money was used to provide 550 housing units for returning veterans.

In 1947, Saskatchewan Reconstruction Housing Corporation was advanced a further $200,000 from provincial coffers to acquire more housing units. Without doubt, the Reconstruction Housing Corporation was doing as it was intended – providing an important social benefit to returning soldiers.

SASKATCHEWAN RECONSTRUCTION CORPORATION

At the 1946 Legislature sitting, the Premier stated, "The Saskatchewan Reconstruction Corporation has been organized in order to assure the province a more equitable share of surplus war assets."

It had been created in May 1945, by Order in Council No. 676 and no legislative debate. The Corporation was given an advance of $600,000. Records show that the Corporation quickly got down to work acquiring war assets from the federal government at 6% of their assessed value. The assets were then sold throughout Saskatchewan at 10% of their assessed value. Records show that a total of 696 buildings were sold: over 300 for veterans housing, 175 for community centers and churches, 66 to school units, 39 to private investors, and 84 to government agencies.

For the fiscal year April 1, 1946 to March 31, 1947, records show that the Corporation made a profit of over $130,000. When the Corporation was wound down on December 31, 1951, its accrued surplus of $395,054 was all transferred to the Finance department. This was a Crown entity that had served a valuable social purpose in re-utilizing war assets to the betterment of Saskatchewan, all while generating a monetary surplus.

- The Saskatchewan Reconstruction Housing Corporation was created in 1945 to assist returning war veterans in finding housing accommodation.
- The Saskatchewan Reconstruction Corporation was also created in 1945 to acquire surplus war assets and sell them at a small financial gain to communities across the province.

19

Fur and Fish

The Douglas government decided to take steps to open up northern Saskatchewan to economic activity.

SASKATCHEWAN FUR MARKETING SERVICE

At the early 1946 Legislative sitting, the Premier stated: "A survey of the trapping lease areas in Northern Saskatchewan has been in progress for some time, which, when completed, will enable the government to place the trapping industry on a sounder basis than has heretofore been the case."

What he did not make clear was that a few months earlier, in October 1945, Order in Council No. 1525 had created the Fur Marketing Service. Prior to its creation, fur trappers and fur ranchers would deliver their furs to one of the many trading depots in northern Saskatchewan where they would receive a price for their furs. The operators of the trading depot would then bear the cost of shipping the furs by rail to the Montreal fur auction. The trading depot operators would also ensure they extracted a profit for themselves. Through it all, the fur trapper was disadvantaged.

The decision to create the Fur Marketing Service streamlined the fur selling process. Under the new Crown structure, trappers of beaver and muskrat were compelled to send their furs to the newly created fur auction in Regina. Other types of animal furs could be sold in other markets at the discretion of the trapper. Fur ranchers of mink were exempt from having to use the Regina auction.

A two-story, purpose-designed building was created in Regina to process and auction off the beaver and muskrat furs. The Montreal fur auction was soon eclipsed by the size and scale of the Regina fur auction. Payment to trappers and ranchers involved an initial payment and a final payment, not unlike the model used by grain elevators to pay farmers. Before long, over 10,000 trappers were sending their beaver and muskrat furs to Regina.

A sum of $55,000 was advanced to pay for construction of the Regina building and to provide working capital. Records show that from its October 1945 inception to March 31, 1946, a profit of $1,642 was made after paying for equipment. For the fiscal year April 1, 1946 to March 31, 1947, a profit of $32,425 was earned. For some unexplained reason, the fiscal year was then shifted from a March 31 end to a September 30 end. For the shortened fiscal period ended September 30, 1947 a profit of $29,175 was recorded. More importantly, the Fur Marketing Service returned $34,000 to the Finance Department.

Commentary from the 1947 Legislature sitting stated, "The Fur Service has one of the most modern, up-to-date fur sale establishments on the continent, located in Regina, where grading, cleaning and sale of furs is carried on in the interests of trappers and fur ranchers. Buyers come from far and wide for the sales. Previously, Saskatchewan trappers and fur ranchers had no such facilities as these. The majority of them have expressed themselves as being more than satisfied with the prices and the service they obtain from this socially-owned project of the Government of Saskatchewan."

At this same sitting, Opposition Leader William Patterson, took aim at the fur entity saying: "Take, for instance, the Fur Marketing Agency; it claims a profit of $1,642. If that was a private operation, it would have paid the City of Regina taxes on the property it occupies of $600; it would have paid a business tax of $560, for a total of $1,160. It had $55,000 advanced to it from the Treasury; it would have paid at least $2,000 in interest on those advances. How much it might have paid the federal government for income or corporation tax, I don't know. Now, if this Fur Marketing Service made $1,642 in the year ending March 31st, 1946, it made $1,160 at the cost of the taxpayers of the City of Regina. All of us who own property in the City of Regina made a little contribution so that the Minister's pet scheme of fur marketing might show a profit of $1,642. All of us, as taxpayers of the Province of Saskatchewan, paid the interest on the $55,000 which this marketing agency was using."

Patterson's comments would be echoed a decade later in the Mossbank debate where the issue of Crown Corporation expenses being shouldered by the taxpayer would be raised. Interest and taxes aside, the Fur Marketing Service would go on to make money and also return money to the Finance department.

For the fiscal year ended September 30, 1948 profits were just over $56,000. For the fiscal year ended September 30, 1949, profits were just over $31,000. This swing in profitability is tied to the fact that fur prices fluctuated on the world market. But through the price ups and downs, the Fur Marketing Service made money. The building and equipment were expanded and improved. By the fiscal year end of September 1949, records show that the government had advanced a cumulative total of $126,000 to the Fur Service. However, the Fur Marketing Service had by that point paid back to Finance a cumulative sum of $119,500.

The mid-1950s saw a major change in the fur industry. The demand for fur-trimmed coats peaked. Coat trends also changed towards shorter lengths. Shorter coats meant less fur was needed. Trappers were not happy at their reduced revenues and they spoke up loudly. In 1955, the *Fur Act* was amended to remove the compulsory requirement of sending beaver and muskrat furs to Regina. Trappers would now be able to sell their furs to whomever they wanted to maximize their revenues.

Records show that by September 1959, the Finance department had received a cumulative total of $384,922 in remittances from the Fur Marketing Service. The question is, had the Liberals been elected in 1944, would they have started a service to help bring more economic activity to northern Saskatchewan?

SASKATCHEWAN FISH BOARD

In the early 1946 sitting, the Premier announced, "Five fish filleting and freezing plants are in operation. A Crown Corporation has been established for the orderly marketing of Saskatchewan fish."

Government budget figures show the total cost of constructing and equipping the fish filleting plant in Lac la Ronge was $41,693. A second plant was built at Beaver Lake. The combined cost of these two plants was approximately $100,000. Each would fillet a minimum of 500,000 pounds of fish per year, while employing from 15 to 20 workers each. A third plant had been purchased at Dore Lake for $25,000 and options to purchase had been exercised for plants at Buffalo Narrows and Big River.

No sooner had these five plants been made operational, than the fish market dynamics began to shift precariously. The US Pure Foods and Drugs Administration (precursor of the modern-day US Food and Drug Administration) imposed strict quality standards on fish imported from Canada. This was no doubt in an effort to protect the US fresh-water fishing industry. These tighter quality standards forced the Fish Board to categorize Saskatchewan lakes as either Class A or Class B lakes. Fish from Class A lakes could be readily certified for sale and exported. Fish from Class B lakes required rigid inspection by US authorities.

The Fish Board decided to mount a marketing campaign aimed at households across the province. The goal was to raise demand for fish by encouraging families to include fish as part of their weekly meal plans. To distribute filleted fish to households, a mail order service was started. In addition, money was spent to establish experimental units in Prince Albert and Meadow Lake for smoking and canning fish. Financial records do not state whether these experiments were successful or not.

Records for the fiscal year ending October 31, 1947, show that the Fish Board sold $376,519 of fish products. But the operational expenses to realize this revenue amounted to $428,857. For fiscal 1947, the Fish Board lost $95,000 after accounting for all costs. To the end of fiscal 1947, a total of $661,650 had been advanced to the Fish Board since its inception. Clearly the fish business was not profitable. The government had a choice: get out of the fish business or put more money into the venture. The decision was made to put more money in.

On the heels of this decision, the fish market in North America continued to shift as reduced import restrictions made more salt water fish varieties available to consumers. To make matters worse, the federal government then decided to allow commercial fishing on Great Slave Lake in the Northwest Territories. This brought an additional 4 million pounds of fish onto the Canadian market.

The decision was made to write off $364,264 of the cumulative advances that had been made to the Fish Board since its inception and assign the organization to the care and control of a new entity, the Fish Marketing Service. The intention was for this new entity was to act as a non-profit, assisting northern fishermen to find a market for their fish. As the verbiage accompanying the financial statements states: "As of May 1, 1949 the Fish

Board ceased attempting to buy and sell fish as a commercial agency that measures its results by profits and losses on financial statements."

However, monetary advances continued to the new non-profit entity. Records show that as of October 1949, $40,000 had been advanced. Fishing was not something that lent itself to government involvement.

In 1945, the Fur Marketing Service was created to streamline the selling and marketing of furs from northern Saskatchewan. Prior to this entity being created, trappers would deliver their furs to privately owned depots where they would be paid prices below market value. The depot operators would send the furs to the Montreal Fur Auction and earn comfortable profits. The Fur Marketing Service made money and the Regina Fur Auction came to eclipse the Montreal Fur Auction in size.

In 1946, the Fish Marketing Board was created to streamline the selling of fish from northern Saskatchewan. What the Douglas government did not see coming was a move by the US government to impose strict quality standards on fish imported from Canada. The demand for fresh water fish was further affected when salt water fish varieties became available to North American consumers. To make matters worse, the federal government decided to allow commercial fishing on Great Slave Lake in the Northwest Territories. The Fish Marketing Board was an economic failure.

20

Trees and Wooden Boxes

SASKATCHEWAN LAKE AND FOREST CORPORATION

The Forest Products Marketing Board (also referred to as the Timber Board) was created in late 1945. At the 1946 Legislature sitting, it was noted, "A complete inventory of our forest resources is being made, and a Forest Products Marketing Board has been established to facilitate the efficient and economical marketing of provincial timber products. An expanded reforestation program is projected, and all forest protection services are being extended and modernized."

A May 1946 Order in Council created the Saskatchewan Lake and Forest Corporation. The earlier-created Forest Products Marketing Board (Timber Board) was then rolled into this new entity.

The Lake and Forest Corporation held the timber cutting rights on the Crown land in the northern part of the province. Records show that by late 1946, it had been advanced a cumulative sum of $1,220,000. In 1947, it used this capital to open six retail lumber yards across the province to make lumber available to the people of Saskatchewan at a retail selling price 10% below the lawful maximum permitted by the federal Wartime Prices and Trade Board. Records show that for fiscal 1947, the Lake and Forest entity made $236,975. Moreover, records show that for fiscal 1947 a total of $195,000 of this gain had been returned to the Finance department. This Crown entity was making money, but it had a way to go to repatriate all that had been advanced to it.

At the early 1948 Legislature sitting, the Opposition was troubled because no depreciation was being accounted for on the financial statements. The Opposition was also angered that the government had opted to provide the people of the province with cheaper lumber instead of exporting lumber to American buyers which would have yielded larger profits.

This concern highlights the difference between the CCF policy and the Liberal policy. The Liberals were focused on profit. The Douglas CCF government was focused on the needs of the people. To the Opposition's point, for the 12 months ended October 1950, only 16% of the lumber sold had been sold to American buyers. In the ensuing years, the amount sold to American buyers would gradually increase, but would peak in 1955 at 47%.

In 1948, the government examined the vast tracts of virgin spruce timber in the Dore and Smoothstone Lakes area (about 80 kms north of Big River). It was decided the best way to exploit this timber would be to establish a modern, government-owned, high-efficiency saw mill. This, rather than allowing private sawmill operators from outside the province the opportunity to harvest the timber.

The fear of having out-of-province operators harvest the timber seems misguided. After all, the government controlled the timber rights and were under no obligation at all to allow out-of-province operators the access to this timber. Nevertheless, the decision was made to proceed with a new, high efficiency mill at Big River. By October of 1950, the Big River project had been advanced $370,000.

The sale of wood products was variable and was impacted by construction demand, and overall economic growth patterns. Consider that for the 12 months ending October 1949, the government sold 48,895 board feet of lumber (a board foot is the industry standard of measure for lumber where one board foot is a piece of lumber 12 inches by 12 inches by 1 inch thick). For the 12 months ending October 1950, the government had sold only 29,462 board feet of lumber. In addition to plank lumber, other wood products being sold included pulp wood (to pulp and paper mills), railway ties, power poles, fence posts, and box wood (sawn wood for making wooden crates).

This sales variability drew fire from the Opposition Liberals who accused the government of sitting on over $1 million of lumber inventory that should have been sold into the market. The Opposition hammered the government on the fact that no interest had been paid to the Finance department on the advanced sums of money. They voiced further disappointment that the lumber yards had paid no money or taxes to the communities they operated in.

What the Opposition overlooked was the fact that despite the variability in sales, money was being made from wood products sales. For example, for the 12 months ended October 1950, the Lake and Forest Corporation paid $242,000 to the Department of Natural Resources, remitted $33,000 in EH&S tax (provincial sales tax), gainfully employed 469 people, and booked a profit of $132,253.

However, the picture would soon change as the Big River mill commenced operations. In anticipation of a 1950 startup, the government had arranged for local logging contractors to provide logs. A contract dispute arose and in the end the government was advised by its legal counsel to pay up and settle the matter. To avoid future such disputes, the government decided to hire its own people to cut logs rather than hiring local contractors. It was soon realized that cutting logs and delivering them to the mill was not an easy task. Meanwhile, the mill itself did not perform as anticipated. Production throughput was low and operating costs were high. For fiscal 1951, the Big River operation lost $32,632. For fiscal 1952, the operation lost $64,792. At the end of fiscal 1952, cumulative advances to the Big River operation totaled $580,000. After fiscal 1952, the results of the Big River operation ceased to be separated out from the overall results of the Lake and Forest Corporation. Results from the Big River operation would be buried in the footnotes of future financial statements.

Eventually, the operational issues at the mill were resolved and overall wood products sales improved. Beyond 1952, footnotes in the financial statements indicate the Big River operation was making profits of near $300,000 each year. While the advances received by the Lake and Forest Corporation from the Finance department rose to a cumulative total of over $3.3 million, by October 1956 a total of $2,864,620 had been remitted back to the Finance department. The payback likely would have been faster, but the government made the decision to deploy some of the operating profits into constructing roads in the northern part of the province. This was deemed to be a social benefit that would open the north to more commerce.

SASKATCHEWAN BOX FACTORY

In 1945, the government took over a box factory in Prince Albert, Saskatchewan. In the 1940s, boxes were not the typical cardboard boxes we see today. In those days, boxes referred to wooden boxes. The factory in Prince Albert made egg crates, butter boxes, meat and fish crates, bee hive boxes, fur stretching frames, and granary doors.

At the February 1946 Legislature sitting, Premier Douglas explained how the box factory had become a Crown Corporation, "The box factory was taken over not because of a quarrel with the employees, but because the employer, who was the manager of it, had refused for a year and a half to bargain with his employees. The Union had been organized for a year and a half, had endeavored to secure an agreement, and the matter was taken to the Labour Relations Board. The manager of the plant along with owner Mr. Sifton Davis (truly a name to conjure with), came before the Board and were asked to state why they would not bargain with the Union. After months of delay, no action was taken. I had no intention to take arbitrary action, neither did my colleagues. We wrote to them and asked them to come in and discuss the matter with us. Mr. Davis asked for more time-another week. We gave him the week, and he used that week to transfer the property from the former shareholders to Mr. Mitchell, the manager, not for $11,000 cash, but for $11,000 back salary that the company owed him. He then fired all his past employees with the object of starting negotiations all over again with the new owner. These men, Mitchell and Davis, defied constituted authority in this province. These men flouted the law when it suited their purpose. The plant was taken over because they worked to set the stage to defy constituted authority. Since the plant has been taken over, the men are being treated as human beings, not as beasts of burden, and Mitchell is now offered $50,000 for the plant he paid $11,000 for as back wages."

At the early 1947 sitting, MLA Procter asked the government the following question: "What was the total amount paid to the former owner of the box factory at Prince Albert for buildings, plant, machinery, equipment, supplies and other materials? Minister Joe Phelps replied, "Stock in trade $12,597.31, land, buildings, machinery and equipment $58,902.60 for a total of $71,500.00." An examination of financial statements indicates that to March 1947, the cumulative sum advanced to the box factory totaled $153,902.

At this same 1947 sitting, Opposition Leader, William Patterson, hammered the government on the subject of depreciation, "Here the government took over not a new business, but a going concern, about November 1, 1945. There was no interruption of operations. As a matter of fact, shortly after the government took over, there were stories about the additional business they were doing, yet in five months they had run up a loss of $7,800! I do not know how much taxes this concern would have paid the City of Prince Albert had it continued to be operated by a private owner, but I do know the box factory claimed depreciation of $1,400 on a total investment of $70,000."

Records show that in 1949 the controversial box factory was shifted to the control of Saskatchewan Lake and Forest Products. This was likely done to divert attention away from future criticism. At the end of 1956, the box factory was sitting on a cumulative deficit of $352,148. It was simply not financially viable. Should it have been taken over by the government in the first place? Was the reasoning for the takeover based on economics? Or was the takeover a strategy to solidify the labour movement in the province?

- In 1945, the Forest Products Marketing Board was established to facilitate the efficient and economical marketing of provincial timber. The government learned that cutting logs and delivering them to a mill for sawing in lumber was not an easy task.
- In 1945 the government acquired a wooden box factory in Prince Albert by way of some unusual circumstances. The cumulative deficit of this venture shows that it was not successful.

21

Airplanes and Buses

SASKATCHEWAN GOVERNMENT AIRWAYS

In a further effort to open the northern part of the province, the government decided to establish an air service. The mandate was to move trappers, furs, mineral prospectors, and members of the general population around the north. In addition, the mandate was to provide an air ambulance service.

Records show that Saskatchewan Airways was created in the summer of 1947 by an Order in Council. Shortly afterwards, advances of $305,500 were made for the purpose of acquiring a fleet of airplanes. From November 1, 1947 to October 31, 1948, the focus was on building hangars in several northern communities and purchasing airplanes. Records show that in the first fiscal year, the organization recorded a net profit of $14.84.

The Opposition seized on this meagre sum. In the 1948 Legislature session, an Opposition MLA pointed an accusing finger and stated, "The government Airways made $14. They've got $300,000 and they made

$14, before interest! And I think they probably had a pretty good year, last year, because you remember the activity there last July in the northern part of Saskatchewan, in the constituencies of Cumberland and Athabaska. You will remember the number of Cabinet Ministers and members of the Legislature who were up there, and how government planes were scurrying here and there and all over. I am sure those trips were all paid for, and they probably very substantially increased the revenue from this operation as compared with what we can expect in the coming year."

Records for the late 1940s through the early 1950s were not locatable in the Legislature library, however, records show that for the fiscal year ending October 1954, the corporation lost $31,868. For the period ending October 1955, it made $44,755. For the period ending October 1956, Saskatchewan Airways made $60,485.

Running an air service is not cheap, nor is it easy. The corporation had a fleet of 22 aircraft and a staff of 94 employees. To the end of October 1956, cumulative advancements from the government totaled $600,000. Meanwhile, the cumulative surplus generated to the end of October 1955 was $119,902. To the end of October 1956, the cumulative surplus paid back to the Finance department was $180,387. The balance sheet shows the depreciated value of aircraft was $263,110 and the depreciated value of hangar buildings at $130,598. Clearly this was a Crown entity that was serving the social good but at a cost to the taxpayer. The question is, did the social good outweigh the financial costs? Would private enterprise have come into the province to provide air service had the government not gotten involved? Would a Liberal government have done anything to open the north using an airplane service?

SASKATCHEWAN TRANSPORTATION COMPANY

This Crown entity was created in January, 1946, using Order in Council No. 168. The mandate of this Crown entity was stated as: "giving the best service possible, operating whenever and wherever possible without loss, and extending services where needed." At the legislative session in early 1946, the Premier, referring to the Order in Council, advised, "More recently, the Saskatchewan Transportation Company has been formed as a Crown Corporation, and will commence operations on April 1, 1946."

Opposition Leader Patterson (likely concerned that this Crown would be a money loser) then reminded Mr. Douglas for the record that, "At the Session, one year ago, $750,000 was voted in as an estimate of the supplementary funding needed for the Saskatchewan Transportation Company." Startup funding, however, would not be the big issue.

In 1945, the Greyhound Bus Company was providing bus service to many towns in Saskatchewan. There were a variety of other smaller private entrepreneurs providing bus and freight service as well. In one fell swoop, the government pushed Greyhound and the others out of the way and announced that the Saskatchewan Transportation Company had arrived on scene. Greyhound was allowed to maintain its Winnipeg to Calgary and Winnipeg to Edmonton routes, both of which passed through the province. The social benefits of forcing Greyhound and other smaller entrepreneurs to abandon business are hard to fathom.

The government exceeded its 1945 startup capital estimate of $750,000. With government advances of $1.1 million, the new Transportation Crown put together a fleet of 51 buses, and established bus depots in Regina and Saskatoon. By March of 1947, a profit of $36,182 was showing.

At the 1947 session, the Opposition made note of the $1,000,000 that had been spent on buses. It also focused on the $25,000 that had been spent creating a lunch counter at the Regina bus terminal. A sarcastic observation was made that the lunch counter was turning a profit of $8,000 while running the buses was losing about $15,000. What the government had not thoroughly considered was the fact that roads in the province were graveled. Heavy bouts of rain or snow could often make roads difficult to navigate. Variable road conditions directly impacted profitability. For fiscal 1955, a profit of $12,248 was made and in fiscal 1956, a profit of $67,906 was made. Despite the earnings variability, the government pressed ahead. Fiscal 1956 records show the government had advanced a cumulative total of $1,900,000 to the Company and additional newer buses had been purchased.

- Saskatchewan Airways was created in the summer of 1947. This Crown entity served the social good, but at a cost to the taxpayer.
- The Saskatchewan Transportation Company was created in 1946. The Greyhound Bus Company had been providing bus service to many towns in Saskatchewan at the time. The government pushed Greyhound out of the way leaving it with only two cross-province routes. By 1956, the government had advanced a cumulative total of $1,900,000 to this Crown. The earnings did not even come close to repaying the advances.

22

Leather Hides, Shoes, and Blankets

SASKATCHEWAN INDUSTRIES

The early decisions of Minister Joe Phelps to get involved in leather tanning, shoe making, and wool weaving would prove controversial.

Saskatchewan Industries was created by Order in Council No. 1126 in July 1946. Its mandate was to carry on the business of the tannery, shoe, and woollen mill products organizations that had been created in the two previous years.

The records do not clearly state when the tannery operation was first created. What is stated, though, is that its initial plans called for tanning 100 cow hides per day. However, reaching this goal in the post-war economy proved difficult. Not only was there a shortage of cow hides, but there was also a shortage of the chemicals needed for the tanning process. Financial statements show that up to February 1946, the government had injected $43,923 into the tannery. This figure would quickly balloon to $142,500. At issue was the steep learning curve that the employees were navigating. These employees had no prior experience with leather tanning. The financial statements for fiscal 1947 describe how "experiments" were done to create better hide finishes, and to handle different types of leather including horse hides.

Aside from the employee learning curve issue, the profitability of the tannery operation was impacted by the fact that other leather tanneries in North America had re-opened; not only to fill gaps in domestic leather demand but to provide leather goods to war-torn Europe and Japan, both of which were being rebuilt. This was no time for a newly founded operation in Regina to be embarking on an experimental learning curve with unskilled employees.

At the end of December 1947, statements show the tannery had received $152,500 in advances but had made a profit of only $394. Yet, more money was pumped in. At the end of 1948, the tannery had received a cumulative advance of $175,500 in the face of a $39,357 loss. Prices of chemicals were rising. The cost of animal hides was increasing.

By the end of fiscal 1949, Saskatchewan Industries concluded the tannery was a failure. The decision was made to shut the operation down for several months while a reorganization was contemplated. The tannery never did re-open. A total of $73,036 in government advances was written off and the tannery operstion was wound down. The question is, should an attempt at entering the hide tanning business ever have been undertaken? Did Minister Phelps even study the supply and demand scenario for leather? Should more study have been undertaken to better understand the process and the availability of chemicals?

A similar story exists for the shoe products entity. In its early going, it was advanced $40,471 for land, buildings, and basic equipment. To the end of 1946, it had been advanced a cumulative total of $124,000. In early 1947, the shoe factory employed a staff of 30 and was producing shoes at the rate of about 200 pairs daily. Machinery to set up the operation had been obtained through the purchase of a shuttered Winnipeg shoe factory. Individual bits of equipment had been sourced from eastern Canada. The total spent on equipment was approximately $100,000. The plan was to expand beyond just shoes to make leather jackets, and other leather goods as soon as more equipment could be found.

The wages of the 30 employees at the operation ranged from 30 to 45 cents an hour. Opposition Leader Patterson levelled some stinging criticism and noted, "We were told that, when these factories were started, the men in the factories would get more money, and the producer would get more money for his leather product. We were told the men were going to be paid more than the mere minimum. We were told the government would gauge its efforts and determine its policies not 'by what other people did, but by what it thought the right and proper thing to do.' Apparently, however, it is quite all right to get employees to work for 30 to 45 cents an hour."

The anticipated demand for shoes and work boots did not materialize. Moreover, footwear styles were changing. The shoes and boots being made had the soles nailed to the leather uppers. The welted style was now coming into fashion where the leather upper was sewn onto the sole. Unfortunately, the equipment for making welted shoes was hard to find. Moreover, the factory did not have the space to get into other lines of leather shoes. Inventories of nailed-sole shoes and boots was rising. Buyers were not placing orders. The loss for fiscal 1948 came in at $32,600. For fiscal 1948, cumulative advances from the government were at $186,000.

By the end of fiscal 1949, it became clear to Saskatchewan Industries that shoemaking was a failure. A total of $82,727 in government advances was written off and the shoe factory was wound down. Should an effort to make shoes ever have been undertaken? Should more market research have been done prior to launching into the shoe business? The assets of the tannery and the shoe factory were moved to the care and control of the Public Works Ministry for eventual sale.

The woollen mill entity was created in 1945 using advances of $475,000. At the February 1946 sitting, MLA Danielson asked the government what products had been manufactured at the woollen mill up to February 1, 1946? The answer was a curt reply of "woollen blankets."

While a true answer, it was certainly vague. At this same 1946 sitting, Opposition Leader Patterson reminded the government that the woollen mill was supposed to have cost $150,000. He said, "So far as we can learn, the cost is now in the neighborhood of twice that amount. We can get no information as to production, or the cost of production, and, strangely, though this government operation has been underway for more than a year, the Minister admits he does not yet have a sales price list. He offered to sell me a pair of his blankets in this House, but when I asked him what the price was, he could not tell me. It has all been a grandstand play."

MLA Danielson then re-stated his original question, this time asking how many woollen blankets had been produced up to February 1, 1946? The answer was, "It is not in the public interest to give this information."

What the government was not willing to engage in was a discussion that would have revealed private enterprise across North America had re-started weaving operations and had moved to erase any wartime supply shortages of blankets. Retailers across Canada had ample inventories of woollen goods. So saturated was the market that several woollen mills across North America were poised to close and were setting up to dump their unsold inventory onto the saturated market.

At the 1947 sitting, Opposition Leader Patterson laid criticism at the feet of the government stating, "When it was announced that the Government was going to operate a woollen mill, we were told that it would pay the wool growers more money for their wool, that it would sell the products of the mill at lower prices, and that it would provide profits for increased social services. There is no figure in the estimates relating to any of these development projects."

At the early 1948 sitting, the Opposition correctly noted that as of the end of 1947, a cumulative total of $590,000 had been advanced to the operation, and that for fiscal 1947 the wool operation had lost over $88,000. The Opposition then called for a complete plant closure.

But, no sooner had the Opposition voiced these concerns than demand for wool products staged a rebound. The government advanced enough money to the operation to purchase six new automatic looms which promised to deliver reduced operating costs.

Once again, the government failed in its due diligence. The promises of the new looms creating reduced operating costs proved fleeting. The uptick in demand that prompted the purchase of the new looms proved transitory. Records for fiscal 1949 show a total of $785,000 had been advanced to the woollen mill operation. By the end of fiscal 1951, the cumulative advances stood at $830,000. The operation was shut down shortly afterwards.

Clearly, the wool business was not something that could stand on its feet in Saskatchewan. Should it have been started in the first place? Why had it been allowed to limp along, losing money, for so long?

- The government's efforts to get involved in the leather tanning business ran headlong into more efficient private-sector tannery operations across Canada. The government advances were written off and the tannery entity was wound down.
- The story of the woollen mill and the shoe factory are the same. Large cumulative losses followed by factory closures.

23

Bricks and Sodium Sulphate

SASKATCHEWAN MINERALS

In 1945, Premier Douglas spoke about the mineral extraction potential in Saskatchewan. He announced, "As an initial step in this direction, my government has purchased a brick manufacturing plant to be used in the development of a clay products industry within the province. This industry is to be developed in conjunction with a post-war construction program."

He said the cost of the equipment had been $150,000 and that the plant would be capable of making 10 million bricks per year and employing 50 men. What he was alluding to was the fact that the government had purchased the assets of International Clay Products in Estevan, Saskatchewan. What he failed to elucidate was that before the plant could be made fully operational, a complete rebuild of its infrastructure was needed. This took up all of calendar year 1945.

The brick plant started operating in 1946. Process difficulties prevented the plant from realizing much output. In 1947, the decision was made to run the plant year-round. Money was spent to winterize the facility, but difficulties were incurred with that task as well. But the winterization effort eventually was eventually completed and the plant began making bricks.

In 1948, Opposition Leader Patterson seized on these early difficulties. He noted that for fiscal 1947 the brick plant had only shown $13 in depreciation. He said, "The Brickyards depreciated the coal and the clay that was taken from it in its operations by $13 last year. It has advances from the Provincial Treasurer of $237,000." He further criticized the efficiency of the brick plant by noting that in the winter of 1947 about $100,000 had been spent to winterize the facility, which apparently did not work well. The Opposition sarcastically asked, "Would it not have been better to find someone who knew something about making bricks to ensure the winterization efforts would be effective"?

At this same Legislature sitting in 1948, Premier Douglas described that the brick plant was operating on an experimental basis, with 40,000 common bricks being turned out per eight-hour day. His choice of the word "experimental" is interesting. What he was effectively saying was that the plant was not operating at an efficient level.

In 1950, in an effort to improve the efficiency of the operation, capital was allocated to the operation to install a tunnel kiln that would allow for a more continuous process flow. But the new kiln did not eliminate the reality that the bricks were susceptible to developing small cracks during drying. It was determined that the cracking was due to the mineral characteristics of the clay being used. To alleviate these cracking issues, clay of a slightly different composition sourced from Eastend, Saskatchewan and Willows, Saskatchewan was hauled to Estevan.

The brick operation was also drawing criticism from private enterprise. Bruno Clayworks (north of Saskatoon) had been established in the 1920s by a private group of investors. As the government-run plant at Estevan ramped up production, the owners of the Bruno operation started to suffer financially. There was not enough room for two brick plants in the province. Moreover, the government was not issuing tenders for brick needed to build new government buildings across the province. The government was, instead, using its own Estevan brick and thereby squeezing out private competition. In 1960, the Bruno plant shut down, never to reopen. The Douglas government never did explain the social benefits of driving a private enterprise competitor out of business.

By 1955, the brick plant was running at capacity, turning out 26,500 tons of brick annually, with a workforce of 51 men. At the end of fiscal 1956, the government had advanced a cumulative total of $650,000 to the brick operation. The plant, however, had been returning surplus money back to the Finance department. The cumulative deficit to the end of fiscal 1956 was $2,806. Finally, by the end of fiscal 1960–14 years after it had started, the brick plant was operating in the black. But the Douglas government had overlooked the trend of the market. The mid-1950s had seen the start of a construction industry trend away from fired-clay brick towards cheaper concrete blocks. Steel and aluminum structural materials were also coming into fashion. Clay bricks would soon be on their way out.

In the late 1940s, it had been discovered that a mineral called sodium sulphate, when added to molten glass, was effective at removing tiny air bubbles from the molten glass, thus making for better quality glass panes.

Fabric makers had also discovered the benefits of sodium sulphate. Adding sodium sulphate to vats containing cotton fibers reduced the electrostatic charges on the fibers and allowed for a more even penetration of dye colorants into the fibers. The result was a better-looking dyed fabric with uniform coloration.

The paper-making industry also discovered that sodium sulphate could be used in its process. Adding the mineral to vats containing pulp slurry initiated a chemical reaction that created sodium sulfide. The sulfide, in turn, reacted with water in the pulp slurry to make sodium hydrosulfide which degraded the lignin in the pulp slurry. The net result was a more efficient pulping and paper making process.

Nature had bestowed a gift on Saskatchewan. In the mid-1940s, sodium sulphate deposits were identified at Chaplin, Saskatchewan and at Bishopric, Saskatchewan (not far from Mossbank). Sodium sulphate extraction got underway at Chaplin in the summer of 1946. (The next time you are driving west on the Trans-Canada highway between Moose Jaw and Swift Current, you will pass by the Chaplin operation with its white mounds of sulphate appearing in sharp contrast to the surrounding terrain)

The Bishopric operation, along with an operation near Alsask, Saskatchewan (Highway 7 west of Kindersley near the Saskatchewan-Alberta border), had been started by a private company called Natural Sodium Products. The gentleman at the helm of this company then identified a lucrative mineral deposit in South America. To raise money to pursue the South American project, he mortgaged the Bishopric and Alsask operations through a bank in New York. When the South American venture failed, he defaulted on the New York mortgage. In 1954, the New York bankers sold the projects to the Saskatchewan government. The assets were folded into the Saskatchewan Minerals Crown entity. The equipment from Alsask was moved to Bishopric where a plant remodeling was undertaken.

By 1956, the government had advanced a cumulative total of $1,085,000 to the Chaplin and Bishopric sulphate operations. In fiscal 1956, these two operations had a combined gross profit of $416,455. After depreciation, net profit was $182,616. The sodium sulphate business was profitable. This explains why to the end of fiscal 1956, a cumulative total of $659,086 had been repatriated to the Finance department. Moreover, the sulphate operations were paying royalties to the provincial Department of Natural Resources. As of the end of fiscal 1956, the cumulative total of these royalties was $287,000. However, the two extraction operations would soon be melded into one.

Records do not show any evidence that the government sought to determine how many years of mining were left at either extraction site. Nor did the government make any effort to estimate how many tons of high grade, medium grade, and lower grade material were extractible. With today's rigidly structured accounting methods, a determination of all these factors would have been required. Once again, the failure to plan and anticipate caught up with the government. Over the following several years, industry began demanding a higher grade of sulphate material; higher than what Nature had deposited at Bishopric. This necessitated the closure of the Bishopric operation. How many more years it took the Chaplin operation to repatriate the balance of start-up funds owing to the Finance Department is not clear.

(If your travels ever take you to Mossbank, in mid-July of each year the town hosts the Old Wives Lake Festival. One of the available attractions is a bus tour of the surrounding area where you will see the remnants of the old Bishopric operation.)

Would a Liberal government have pursued sodium sulphate operations? Would they have pursued brick making to satisfy the demands for construction brick? Perhaps the bigger question is, why did the government aggressively pursue brick operations when the privately owned Bruno, Saskatchewan plant was already well established? Where were the social benefits? Where were the social benefits of ploughing money into sodium sulphate?

- In the late 1940s, it was discovered that a mineral called sodium sulphate proved beneficial for manufacturers of glass windshields, for manufacturers of dyed cotton fabric, and for the pulp and paper industry. In the mid-1940s, sodium sulphate deposits were identified at Chaplin, Saskatchewan and at Bishopric, Saskatchewan (not far from Mossbank). The grade of sulphate being extracted at Bishopric eventually proved unsatisfactory to industry and the facility was shuttered, leaving only the Chaplin operation in production.
- In 1945, the government purchased a brick making plant. The government overlooked the trend in the construction industry¬ – a shift away from fired clay fired bricks towards cheaper concrete blocks. This failure to read the market, to plan and to anticipate caught up with the government.

24

Horses, Printing, and Radio

HORSE COOPERATIVE MARKETING ASSOCIATION LIMITED

A horse meat operation was set up near Swift Current in 1945. The operation is mentioned in the 1945 Legislature proceedings as having been given a government guaranteed loan from the Bank of Montreal for $113,800 with interest of $686.18 for a total owing of $114,486. Also at the 1945 sitting, Premier Douglas noted, "My government has given assistance to the Saskatchewan Co-operative Horse Marketing Association in setting up a processing plant in the province. Special study is being given to the industrial uses of the by-products of the industry." Government budget data suggests about 100 horses were being slaughtered per day using a workforce of 60 men. There was a $5 million contract with the Belgian government to provide horse meat for human consumption with process by-products being sold to fur ranching operations as feed for mink and muskrat. Government records do not indicate how many years this operation continued for.

Saskatchewan Government Printing

At the 1946 Legislature sitting, Minister Fines stated, "Since March of 1945, the government has owned and operated a modern printing plant in Regina, which has been turning out printing at the rate of about $100,000 a year, at a saving of 20 per cent."

This operation had been created by Order in Council No. 859 in June 1945. The mandate was to provide printing services to the various government departments.

In 1947, the printing entity drew Opposition fire when MLA Patterson said, "The printing plant shows a very substantial margin of profit. It, too, enjoys the benefits that I have already explained: no federal taxation; no city taxation. In addition to that it enjoys the advantage (a very material one for a business) that the government can feed it all the business it can take all the time. It does not have to worry about any slack period, or anything of that kind. Now it claims to have made a profit of $6,400. Well, the people of Regina, the taxpayers of Regina, those of us who happen to own property in Regina and pay the taxes to keep this city going, we contributed $1,460 of that, indirectly, because, if that had been a private business, that is the amount it would have paid into the coffers of the city; and because it did not pay it, the rest of us had to make it up."

Mr. Patterson was correct in his profit margin statement and in his observations about not paying taxes. The tax issue had been forced onto the shoulders of the taxpayers of Regina. But the printing operation with its 50 employees was handily making money. By the end of fiscal 1956, the operation had remitted back to Finance the sum of $469,937. Clearly printing was a money maker. But it had a captive audience. Government departments had no choice but to direct their printing through this plant. And true to Patterson's 1947 observation, as of 1956, there were still no line items on the financial statements to indicate payment of taxes.

SASKATCHEWAN RADIO BROADCASTING CORPORATION

At the 1946 sitting, Opposition Leader Patterson asked Finance Minister Fines if the government had created a radio broadcasting corporation and when it became operational. Fines replied, "Yes, on January 25, 1946." Details in budget records are scarce and there are no financial statements at the Legislature library. If such a Crown entity ever was established, it appears that it did not undertake any acquisitions or exist very long.

- In 1945, at attempt was made to start a horse meat operation near Swift Current. Records do not indicate how much start-up capital was advanced to the project, or if it even managed to commence operations.
- In 1945, a government printing office was created. Clearly this was a money maker. But it had a captive audience – government departments that had no choice but to direct their printing through this plant.
- In 1946, the government apparently advanced funds to start a radio broadcasting entity. No financial records could be located.

25

Insurance

SASKATCHEWAN GOVERNMENT INSURANCE CORPORATION

The *Saskatchewan Government Insurance Act,* was passed by the Douglas government in 1946. At the same time, the *Automobile Accident Insurance Act* was also passed.

These two Acts imparted a dual responsibility to the government. The government was to administer general insurance in nearly every category, and sell it to Saskatchewan residents at a low cost. Secondly, the government was to collect auto insurance premiums and use the premiums to pay accident claims and to cover the operating costs of administering the claims service.

The general insurance categories authorized were: (a) fire insurance; (b) life insurance; (c) automobile insurance; (d) accident insurance; (e) aircraft insurance; (f) boiler and machinery insurance; (g) guarantee insurance;

(h) inland transportation insurance; (i) live-stock insurance; (j) plate glass insurance; (k) property damage insurance; (l) public liability insurance; (m) sickness insurance; (n) theft insurance, and (o) weather insurance.

The *Saskatchewan Government Insurance Act* called for the creation of the Saskatchewan Government Insurance Office, to be run by a manager and overseen by the Minister. The Act stated that people could become agents to sell insurance on behalf of the Government Insurance Office. Annual fees to act as an agent for all classes of insurance were $25 in a city, $7 in a town, and $3 elsewhere.

The *Automobile Accident Insurance Act* stipulated the creation of an Auto Fund that would collect and disburse insurance premiums as required.

The Saskatchewan Government Insurance Corporation was created to administer both 1946 Acts. A total of $12,000 was advanced to start the operation. The social motivation to start this Crown structure was the fact that from April 1, 1946 through December 31 1947, 2,728 persons were killed or injured in the province in automobile accidents. Moreover, a Crown entity to engage in the selling of insurance to Saskatchewan residents cheaper than they could buy it from private enterprise was not only socially responsible, it stood to be a money maker as well. To illustrate how profitable the insurance business could be, in the period April 1, 1947 through December 31, 1947 the Insurance Office wrote $620,102 in premiums and only paid out $241,853 in claims.

Despite the money being made, the government was nebulous in its disclosure of details pertaining to the Insurance operation. At the 1946 Legislature sitting, Opposition Leader Patterson asked the government about the rates of commission being paid to agents selling insurance for the Saskatchewan Government Insurance Office. The blunt response was, "It is not in the public interest to state the rates." At this same sitting, Mr. Patterson asked the government about the total premium charged by the Saskatchewan Government Insurance Office for a five-point automobile policy on a privately owned and operated, Chevrolet 1942 model automobile? The blunt answer was," $18.50", with no details added.

By 1955, the Insurance Office employed 329 people and had purchased its own building in Regina. Its investments on its Balance Sheet were listed at over $8 million.

Insurance accounting is somewhat difficult to follow. How it works is the gains made from the automobile insurance part of the business are taken up by the Auto Fund, which in itself has a significant sum of investments.

For example, consider the 1955 fiscal year. The automobile insurance part of the operation made a gain of $2,170,550 on $5,636,470 of premiums written.

The Auto Fund then siphoned off this underwriting gain of $2,170,550 and inserted it into its own profit and loss statement. At the end of December 1954, the Auto Fund had been sitting on a surplus of $490,812. Adding the 1955 surplus of $2,203,645 to the pot brought the Auto Fund profit surplus to $2,300,233.

For 1955, the general insurance part of the operation showed an underwriting gain of $118,992. The Government Insurance Crown entity was proving itself a money maker. Records show that to the end of fiscal 1956, a cumulative total of $2,291,545 of surpluses had been remitted to Finance.

In a review of Legislative proceedings beyond 1949, a lessening of Opposition critique of the Crown Corporations is noticeable. Oil, potash, and minerals had all been discovered in Saskatchewan. Schools and hospitals were being constructed. Highways were being built. The economic picture in the province was improving. The Opposition had many more things to critique and their focus shifted away from the Crowns.

- In 1946, the government entered the insurance business. Despite some occasional peculiarities in its accounting disclosures, this Crown entity did make money, and continues today.

26

Telephones and Power

Lastly, the array of Crown Corporations includes telephones and power. However, these were not created by the Douglas government.

SASKATCHEWAN TELEPHONE CORPORATION

Saskatchewan Telephone Corporation was established with the passing of the *Telephone Act* on June 12, 1908. Initially, the company was known as the Department of Railways, Telegraphs and Telephones. It grew by acquisition of other independent telephone companies (including the Bell Telephone Company of Canada's Saskatchewan operations), and quickly became the dominant telephone operator in Saskatchewan. The new company was funded through the issuance of long-term Saskatchewan government debentures bearing an interest rate of 4%. The 1908 Legislative proceedings describe that, "the Lieutenant Governor in Council shall have power to authorize the Provincial Treasurer from time to time to issue debentures of the province in sums not exceeding one thousand dollars, each bearing interest at a rate not exceeding four per cent per annum and payable at any time not exceeding forty years from the date thereof."

In the early 1929 legislative proceedings, questions were raised concerning whether the Telephone Company was remitting surpluses to the government. The Minister's response was, "On page 23 of the Public Accounts will be found the sum of $280,000 paid to the province as repayment of capital. In the Department of Telephones, it has been the practice from time to time to repay to the Provincial Treasury sums of money which go into the sinking fund and are used for the redemption of debentures issued for the Department."

Telephones were a money maker for the government. This situation would continue into the future. During 1948, government records show 7,000 new telephone installations which brought the total number of installations in the province to 64,322. Long distance calls, which numbered 4.2 million in 1947, increased to near 4.5 million during 1948.

By 1949, Saskatchewan Telephones was officially being labeled as a success story. At the 1949 sitting, Finance Minister Fines noted that for fiscal 1948, "An examination of the statements show that Telephones has earned $1,608,000 on total average advances of $8,793,000, before interest." In percentage terms, Saskatchewan Telephones was earning 18% per year before interest.

SASKATCHEWAN POWER

Saskatchewan Power was founded by the Liberal government as the Saskatchewan Power Commission in February 1929. Initial progress was slow. The vast geographic expanse of the province was dotted with small rural villages. Many of these villages were generating their own electricity using a steam engine that powered a generator. This reality provided little incentive to the government to spend money stringing lines and poles across the province.

The metric used to gauge power distribution was the *load factor*. The load factor refers to the cost of keeping a distribution line fully charged and to the amount of electricity consumed at the terminal end of a distribution line. In 1929, Jimmy Gardiner's Minister responsible for the Power Commission pointed out, "The greatest problem which the electrical engineer has to face today is the problem of rural electrification. Transmission lines are costly things. Before any rural community can be served, the high line has to feed first some urban centre in the community where the consumption of electricity is sufficient to justify the cost of transmission line and transformers, and take care of line losses together with the keeping of the line energized for twenty-four hours while the demand upon it is only during a very small part of that time; in other words, where the load factor is poor. It is all nonsense to talk about a comprehensive scheme of rural electrification, just now."

The Minister then further reinforced the idea that it might be best to leave rural electrification in the hands of individual municipalities. Citing the Alberta situation, he said, "In Alberta, most of the distribution is in the hands of the municipalities, who buy their power from private companies and then retail the power to consumers. In some cases, the municipalities have generating power plants of their own. The Public Utilities Commission exercises control over rates. It may be said that, in Alberta, the private companies have the right of way."

In fact, the private model was creeping into Saskatchewan as well. In a lengthy speech given in February 1929, E.S. Wheatly, the Conservative MLA for Kindersley, said, "As I see it, from the report of the Commission, our resources of power in the north and south are too far removed from the great centres of population, and this militates against the construction of power lines in an economic way. Possibly, therefore, there will have to be a period of marking time. Now, it seems to me this marking time is not a good thing, and, as has been stated in this House, something over 100 franchises have been taken over by private interests. To my mind, that is going to complicate things seriously when the government does start out, and to my mind, something should be done. As I say, the encroachments of these private interests into the field of power in this province, are not reassuring."

He concluded by urging the government to buy some of these private operators, "They are here, as I say, to make money and are not going to operate in the interests of the people. So, I say, if we are going into power, why not step out now? When these franchises are for sale, would it not be better to buy them up now? We might not have our scheme ready; we might not be able to include them in the network of comprehensive power lines, but if it is going to pay these private interests, would it not pay us as a government to take these up and conduct them until such time as we are able to incorporate them in a provincial scheme?"

When the Douglas CCF government took the reins of power, the hesitating came to an end. A strategy of buying out private power operators was put into play. In March 1945, Resources Minister Joe Phelps explained that in 1944, "The Saskatchewan Power Commission, on behalf of the Crown in the right of the province, agreed to purchase the entire common stock of Dominion Electric Power Limited, subject to the passing of legislation to authorize the Commission to make the purchase, and subject to the passing of any Order in Council required under the provisions of the legislation. The closing date, on which the stock will be transferred and the price paid, will be subsequent to the passing of such legislation and Order in Council."

The purchase price for Dominion Electric's operations at Estevan was $420,000, financed through a bank loan. Another big purchase quickly followed. At this same March legislative sitting, Minister Phelps went on to explain, "Late the same year, we bought another large power company, Prairie Power Company Limited, at a price of $1,462,000 cash. These companies were taken over by the government as a means of expanding and coordinating the services offered by the Saskatchewan Power Commission. It is hoped eventually to provide vastly improved power services to Saskatchewan residents. The Power Commission now owns 2,486 miles of transmission lines compared with 1,626 miles a year ago, and has 24,627 services compared with 12,989 services a year ago."

Saskatchewan Power continued to grow and expand. At the 1946 sitting, Premier Douglas noted, "During the past year, there has been considerable expansion in the activities of the Saskatchewan Power Commission. By purchase and extension of existing lines the number of customers served by the Commission has been almost doubled." He went on to note, "A further step in the government's program of ownership of public utilities was taken when the entire Saskatchewan holdings of Canadian Utilities Limited were purchased by the province. With the exception of one private company and a few isolated units, the electric power industry in the province is now under public ownership."

Government budget figures confirm the progress made between 1944 and 1946: at December 31,1944 there was 1,626 miles of transmission line and at December 31, 1946 there was 2,651 miles, an increase of 1,051 miles. In 1944, 146 towns and villages had been electrified. This number had reached 255 by the end of 1946.

In 1947, Opposition Leader Patterson offered words of praise for both Saskatchewan Power and Saskatchewan Telephones. It seems he found these Crown entities to be good stewards of money. "The Provincial Treasurer tells us that the people of Saskatchewan are the shareholders in these corporations. Well, on that basis, they have been the shareholders in the Telephone Department and the Power Commission for many years; but on any money that has been advanced to those organizations, or those activities, the interest which it would cost the Provincial Treasury has been repaid by those particular activities, and you can say, by and large, that over all of the years every nickel or every cent that the Telephone Department or the Power Commission has cost the province, or the people of the province, by reason of money advanced to them has been repaid."

In 1947, 690 farms were connected to power lines and in 1948, 985 more were connected. In 1948, Saskatchewan Power generated 312,865,000 kilowatt hours, an increase of 9.4 % over 1947, and an increase of 87% over 1939. By 1948 the Power Commission owned 4,190 miles of transmission line serving some 51,000 customers, compared with 1,626 miles of transmission line serving 13,000 customers in 1944.

By 1949, Saskatchewan Power was also being labeled as a success story. At the 1949 sitting, Finance Minister Fines noted, "The Power Corporation earned $1,125,655 before interest is provided, on total advances of $20,184,000, a return of 5.6%."

- The Saskatchewan Telephone Corporation was established in 1908. During 1948 alone, 7,000 new household telephone installations were made bringing the province-wide total to 64,322.
- For fiscal 1948 the Telephone Corporation earned $1,608,000 on advances of $8,793,000 (an 18% return).
- Saskatchewan Power Commission in February 1929. In 1929, Jimmy Gardiner's Minister responsible for the Power Commission pointed out, "It is all nonsense to talk about a comprehensive scheme of rural electrification, just now." This opened the way for private electrical generation operations to start creeping into the province. When the Douglas CCF government took the reins of power, a strategy of buying out private power operators was put into play.
- For fiscal 1948, the Power Corporation earned $1,125,655 before interest on total advances of $20,184,000 (a 5.6% return).

27

Accounting Basics

The previous chapters describing the various Crown Corporations contain references to items like interest payments and depreciation. This chapter briefly describes these basic accounting principles for the benefit of readers who do not regularly encounter such terms.

ABC PRIVATE COMPANY BALANCE SHEET (YEAR 1)

A Balance Sheet is a snapshot of the financial conditions of a company at a given moment in time. The Balance Sheet is divided into three sections: *Assets*, *Liabilities*, and *Equity*. Assets are the investments and equipment items that the company owns. Liabilities are what the company owes to creditors. The net difference between Assets and Liabilities is Equity, which is the net worth of the company.

Consider the following example:

A group of investors decides to start the ABC company. They pool together $100,000 cash with which to start the venture. The company purchases some equipment with the cash. The company also takes out a five-year bank loan of $20,000 at an interest rate of 5%. The Balance Sheet at the time the ABC company started doing business would appear as follows:

Assets
Cash: $40,000
Equipment: $80,000
Liabilities
Bank Debt: $20,000
Equity
$100,000

ABC PRIVATE COMPANY PROFIT AND LOSS STATEMENT (YEAR 1)

A *Profit and Loss Statement* shows the money earned by the company for an accounting period (either a calendar quarter or a calendar year) along with the various expenses made by the company.

ABC Company uses its equipment to manufacture consumer goods which it then sells. Over time, equipment wears out, loses its value, and needs to be replaced. This is reflected on both the Balance Sheet and the Profit and Loss statement through an item called *Depreciation*. Suppose the $80,000 of equipment is expected to wear out and be worthless in eight years. The ABC Company decides the equipment will be depreciated at a rate of $10,000 per year.

In the first 12 months of business, loan repayments are $4529. A Profit and Loss statement for these first 12 months of business operation would look like the following:

Goods Sold: $47,000
Cost of Goods Sold: $20,000

General Expenses: $15,000
Loan Repayments: $4529
Gross Profit: $7,471
Depreciation: $10,000
Taxable Income: ($-2529)
Taxes: $0
Net: ($-2529)

ABC PRIVATE COMPANY BALANCE SHEET (YEAR 2)

After the first 12 months of operations, the ABC Company takes its gross profit of $7,471 and adds it to its Balance Sheet. The depreciation is displayed as a line item called Accumulated Depreciation. The bank debt has been paid down to $16,388. ABC's Equity now stands at $101,083. This is slightly higher than when the company was started because of no taxation on the net loss.

Assets
Cash: $47,471
Equipment: $80,000
Accumulated Depreciation: ($10,000)
Liabilities
Bank Debt: $16,388
Equity
$101,083

As I studied the various financial reports for Crown Corporations from the 1940s and 1950s, I soon learned that government accounting expresses numbers slightly differently. Let's take this ABC Company example and look at it through the lens of government. For ease of comparison, this government example has been kept fairly close to the ABC Private Company example.

The government decides it wishes to create the ABC Crown Corporation.

The Finance department provides ABC with $120,000 from general government coffers. The government then also provides a loan to ABC that has been raised by the Finance department selling five-year government bonds at a 5% coupon rate to investment banks in Toronto and New York. The money raised is used in part to buy some equipment which will be used to manufacture consumer goods which will be sold.

ABC CROWN BALANCE SHEET (YEAR 1)

The Balance Sheet as ABC starts doing business would appear as follows:

> **Assets**
> Cash: $40,000
> Equipment: $80,000
> **Liabilities**
> Deficit: $20,000
> **Surplus**
> $100,000

Note that the term Bank Debt has been replaced with the term *Deficit*. Note that the term Equity has been replaced with the expression *Surplus*.

Over time, ABC's equipment wears out, loses value, and needs to be replaced. This is reflected on both the Balance Sheet and the Profit and Loss statement by way of a Depreciation line item. Suppose the equipment is expected to wear out and be worthless in eight years. It will be depreciated at an arbitrary rate dictated by someone in the bureaucracy.

ABC CROWN PROFIT AND LOSS STATEMENT (YEAR 1)

A Profit and Loss statement for the first 12 months of business operation would look like the following:

Goods Sold: $47,000
Cost of Goods Sold: $20,000
General Expenses: $15,000
Gross Profit: $12,000
Depreciation: $2,000
Surplus that can be Repaid to Finance: $10,000

Note that there is no line item for debt repayment. The government certainly owes interest payments on the bonds that were sold to investment bankers, but the ABC Crown entity bears no responsibility for these interest payments. That responsibility falls on the shoulders of the taxpayer and the general government coffers; a pattern evident in the Crown Corporation financial statements from the 1940s and 1950s.

The government (if it so choses) can make the argument that the ABC Crown has generated a return of $10,000 on the $120,000 of initial funding for a return of 8.3%.

If a depreciation of $0 was used, the surplus would be $12,000 for a return of 10%.

This example of government accounting will also assist you in understanding the nature of some of the debate arguments from 1957. Mr. Thatcher insinuated that under the Douglas government, many of the Crown Corporations were not following generally accepted accounting standards. Depreciation did not follow a defined schedule. Loans and advances received from the Finance department carried no defined repayment schedule. Interest on these loans and advances was not paid.

But the Douglas government did not invent the idea of not following a defined depreciation schedule. In 1936 well before the Douglas CCF government was formed, William Patterson, Liberal Premier and Treasurer, admitted, "As in former years, no, provision has been made for depreciation on the items 'Public Buildings and Public Improvements,' nor for losses which may, and invariably will occur, in the realization of Loans and Advances to Provincial Boards and Commissions."

28

Game On in Mossbank

As Thatcher was demeaning Premier Douglas and the Saskatchewan Crown Corporations, Douglas pulled a page from his political playbook. In a speech in Ogema, Saskatchewan, he described Thatcher as "a liar and a traitor." Thatcher was made aware of what Douglas had said. Evidently, Thatcher's House of Commons comments had rankled Premier Douglas. With neither side willing to back down, it was agreed that the best course of action would be to have Thatcher and Douglas debate each other; anywhere, anytime. This is exactly what Ross Thatcher wanted–a chance to express his opinions at a high-profile event in front of a crowd of voters.

The agreement to debate Thatcher was classic Tommy Douglas–more concerned about the greater good than himself. Douglas did not have to agree to a debate. He could have sat in the comfort of his Regina home and watched the federal election unfold around him. He knew Hazen Argue was a skilled CCF politician who could stand up for himself in the race for the riding of Assiniboia.. Instead, Tommy Douglas threw himself into the fray, seeking to protect the ideals of the Crown Corporation structures that Mr. Thatcher had so vehemently criticized.

The two men agreed that the debate would take place on May 20, 1957, a mere three weeks before the June 10 election date. For the event venue, Thatcher chose the tiny farming village of Mossbank, Saskatchewan located on the northern edge of the Assiniboia riding. It was game on. Thatcher versus Douglas.

MOSSBANK

The Town of Mossbank is located in Rural Municipality 102, Township 11, Range 30 West of the 2nd Meridian. Drive 68 kilometers south-southwest from Moose Jaw on Highway 2 and look for the exit sign into Mossbank. For the more technologically astute, the GPS coordinates are 49.94N, 105.96W.

Mossbank is situated a couple miles south of an alkaline lake called Lake Johnston (more commonly called Old Wives Lake). How did these two names come about?

Around 1840, a massive fire swept across the prairies. The fire drove the buffalo herds westward. A group of Cree Indians from the Qu'Appelle area trekked west to hunt these migrating buffalo. They eventually found a large herd grazing near a large alkaline lake. But the Cree were now in Blackfoot territory. The Blackfoot made a cursory attack on the hunting party, leaving several Cree wounded. A second attack the next morning was anticipated and a group of elderly Cree women offered to remain behind while the rest of the hunting party made haste to trek back to Qu'Appelle under cover of darkness. All night long, the women tended the fires. Blackfoot scouts, seeing the burning fires believed the entire Cree hunting party was still camped there. The next morning when the Blackfoot made their attack, all they found was a small group of old women. Angered at being tricked, the Blackfoot massacred the elderly Cree women. The name *Old Wives Lake* is a reference to this morbid historical event.

In 1872, the Government of Canada acquired the western land holdings of the Hudson Bay Company. In the 1880s, a British aristocrat desperately wanted to see these western lands. After arriving in Canada, he took the train to Moose Jaw. He was then accompanied by a group of North West Mounted Police officials on a trek south of Moose Jaw through the Dirt Hills. He was apparently impressed at the sight of a large lake in the midst of the prairie. The British aristocrat was Mr. Johnston and the lake now also bears his name.

The Dominion Land Act of 1872 created the framework for homesteading in western Canada. The area around Lake Johnston started to attract settlers. A person wishing to homestead could "enter" a quarter-section of land for a fee of $10 payment. The claimant had to reside on the quarter section for at least six months in each of the following three years and cultivate at least ten acres of land per year for each of these three years. The claimant also had to be a British subject by birth or by naturalization.

A Post Office was opened on September 15, 1909 at the home of Mr. Robert Jolly (Section 12, Township 11, Range 30, West 2nd). When traveling south on Highway 2, drive 2.7 kilometers past the first exit into Mossbank. Near the railway tracks, on the west side of the road you will spot a historical stone cairn marking where Mr. Jolly had his Post Office.

Mr. Jolly was a homesteader from Kirkenbright, Scotland. It is not entirely clear how Mr. Jolly arrived at the name Mossbank for the post office location. History books simply state that he coined the expression Mossbank, which was his right to do as Postmaster at the time.

In 1913, a settlement was started just north and east of the Jolly residence. A store owned by Lawrence Quinn started selling goods to local settlers.

On February 14, 1914, the Post Office at the Jolly residence was moved to Mr. Quinn's store. The name Mossbank followed along to the new settlement.

The move of the Post Office to Quinn's store was triggered by competing railway developments. In 1913, the CNoR (Canadian Northern Railway– the precursor of modern day CNR) had arrived in the area by way of Mitchellton and Ardill. The CNoR tracks then went on down to Assiniboia and surrounding area.

In 1914, Canadian Pacific Railroad (CPR) arrived in the area by way of the towns of Dunkirk and Expanse. The CPR tracks then went on to Vantage and points thereafter. The CPR purchased a portion of land from a Mr. Ed Brink and proceeded to establish a townsite called Reycraft. The history books are unclear, but it seems that the old Reycraft townsite would have been roughly where the South Country Equipment dealership is located in Mossbank today.

With the arrival of the CPR, a number of businesses sprung up in Reycraft: Bert Anderson opened a livery and feed stable, Phil Rawlinson started a hardware store, Ed Brink opened a restaurant, a Mr. Urquhart opened a private bank, a Mr. van Tassel opened a pool hall, a Mr. Agar opened a garage, Al Stark opened a harness shop, Bob Foote opened a butcher shop, Alf Wyldman opened a print shop and newspaper, Ross McLaughlin opened a drugstore, a Norwegian church was started, two lumber yards were established, and the Orange Lodge opened.

Two small settlements immediately adjacent to one another was not practical. An opinion in favour of combining the two small settlements started to gather momentum. There were some settlers in the area who had come from Fosston, Minnesota. They argued that a combined settlement should be called Fosston. However, after much heated discussion, the name Mossbank prevailed. Business owners soon skidded their Reycraft buildings over to the Mossbank site. On December 14, 1915, the village of Mossbank was incorporated.

It was eventually decided that Mossbank needed a community hall. A Mr. E.A. Bodie spearheaded the efforts and local residents purchased equity shares in the project. Other residents acquired shares by donating their time and labour. Lumber was salvaged from old grain elevators in the villages of Willowbunch and Willows. At one point, a raffle was held for a new car as a means of raising money for the project. In 1946, records show that the village of Mossbank bought stock in the Community Hall for a total of $500.

Little else is mentioned about the Hall in council minutes until 1953 when a Mr. Lorne Sadlemeyer was granted a license to operate a bowling alley and a pool room in the basement.

It was this Mossbank Community Hall that was selected as the location for the debate event between Thatcher and Douglas. It is not stated in the history books exactly why Ross Thatcher chose Mossbank. Perhaps because it was the closest community to Moose Jaw with a building large enough to host a sizeable public event. Or, perhaps by picking a place close to Moose Jaw, members of the media would be more inclined to attend. What is known for sure is that local residents Cal Suttor, Jean Bouree, Alex Mitchell, and Gravelbourg MLA Lionel Coderre were solidly behind the venue and worked together to decorate the inside of the Hall with Liberal posters in preparation for the event.

The media did indeed come: CHAB Radio from Moose Jaw and CBC Radio from Regina. Moreover, people came; by the hundreds. Some accounts suggest there were close to 1000 people in attendance. The moderator of the debate was Dr. F.H. Wigmore, after whom the present-day hospital in Moose Jaw is named. Fred Wigmore had been born in Prince Edward Island in 1907. He initially studied Theology at Mount Allison University in New Brunswick. Along the way, he was convinced to switch to Medicine. He completed his medical studies at Dalhousie University in Halifax and then his surgery residency in Toronto. After serving in the war, he moved to Saskatchewan and started a medical practice. But Dr. Wigmore had not the first choice for moderator. That distinction had initially been offered to Father Athol Murray, founder of the famed Notre Dame boys' school in Wilcox, Saskatchewan. But when the archbishop in Regina found out that Murray was going to dabble in a political event, he stepped in front of Murray, telling him to forget the idea. In need of a well-known personality, the debate organizers turned to Dr. Wigmore.

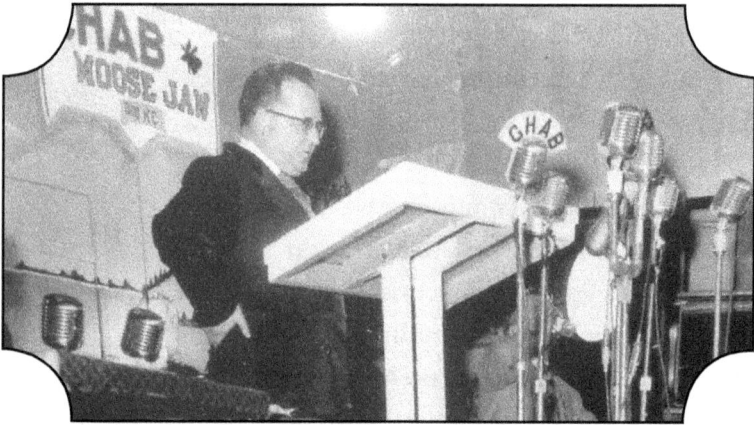

Ross Thatcher Drives Home His Point

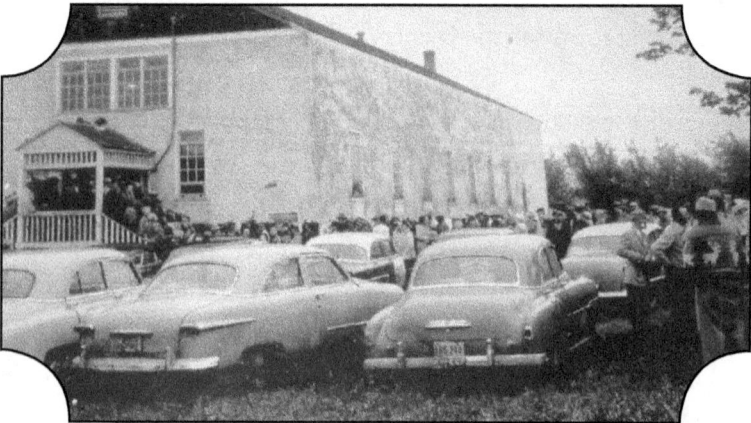

Debate attracts media and spectators to the crowded community hall

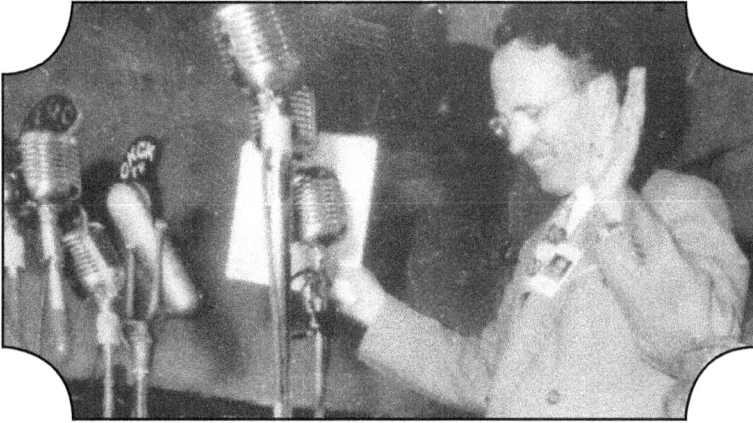

Tommy Douglas defends his Crown Corporations

- After demeaning Premier Douglas and the Saskatchewan Crown Corporations in speeches in the House of Commons, Thatcher got the result he was looking for–a debate. This is exactly what Ross Thatcher wanted – a chance to express his opinions at a high-profile event in front of a crowd of voters.
- The agreement to debate Thatcher was classic Tommy Douglas– more concerned about the greater good than himself. Douglas did not have to agree to a debate. He could have sat in the comfort of his Regina home and watched the federal election unfold around him.

29

The Debate

The following is the transcript of the 1957 debate that took place at the Mossbank Community Hall. This transcript was obtained from Saskatchewan NDP Leader, Carla Beck, whose staff members sourced it from the Archives of Saskatchewan. In preparing this chapter, liberty was taken to correct grammatical errors.

Mr. Chairman: Ladies and Gentlemen. I am sure you are all waiting anxiously and patiently for the commencement of this debate on the record of the Saskatchewan Crown Corporations. Before you have the pleasure of listening to the two gentlemen who are engaged in this debate, it is in order for the Chairman to tell you that the debate will be conducted under the rules and regulations of parliamentary procedure and according to the rules that have been generally adopted to govern all regulated public debates.

It is not necessary that I enumerate all these rules and regulations for either of these speakers, with their long record of public office, but for the benefit of this listening audience, who may not be so familiar with and used to these procedures, I am going to point out certain rules of order and rules of debate.

Neither speaker may refer to the other by his name. Each speaker must adhere to the subject under discussion. No discourteous or personal remarks may be made. No one may interrupt the speaker, except on a point of order and all remarks must be addressed to the chair. The audience may applaud, but heckling in any form, is not permissible.

It is the duty of the Chairman to see that these rules are followed and that fair hearing is given to each speaker. I believe this audience is fair minded and I ask you to give each speaker your close attention.

I do not anticipate that either of these speakers, or the audience, will deviate from what they know to be good conduct, but if either do, I shall not hesitate to fulfill the duties of a Chairman.

The first speaker, the Premier of Saskatchewan, will open the debate and will have 40 minutes to present his case. I shall warn him when there is one minute left to go by flashing a red light once. When the flasher stays on, his attention will be drawn to the fact that his time is up.

The second speaker, the Liberal candidate for Assiniboia, will be given 40 minutes to present his case and he will be warned in a like manner but the red light will be turned off for a further ten minutes, during which time he may make his rebuttal.

The first speaker will then close the debate in a ten minute period. He will be warned in the same fashion.

Ladies and gentlemen, it is my pleasure to ask the Premier of Saskatchewan to open this debate.

Mr. Douglas: Mr. Chairman, Mr. Thatcher, Ladies and Gentlemen.

I want to welcome you all to this debate here in Mossbank tonight. Mr. Thatcher and I just shook hands before we came onto the platform. I don't want anyone to misinterpret that gesture. We shook hands for the same reason as the fellow who was holding hands with his wife. His friend said to him – "You and your wife have been married for 30 years, what are you holding hands for?" He said, "If I don't hold hands with her, she is liable to sock me one."

I want it clearly understood at the beginning, that this debate is being confined to Saskatchewan's Crown Corporations at the insistence of my opponent tonight. I notice the *Regina Leader Post* has a cartoon suggesting that we ought to widen the terms of this debate to general federal issues. I would like to say right here and now that if Mr. Thatcher will say the word, I am prepared to throw this speech away and to discuss federal issues and to prove, I think, to the satisfaction of this audience, that the Liberal government, and particularly Mr. C.D. Howe and Mr. Jimmy Gardiner, have brought western agriculture to the verge of bankruptcy.

I heard some booing. I think this is some of the sheep that Jimmy Gardiner paid $100,000 for. Well, the booing seems to be continuing. I have a stopwatch here, and if it continues....

Spectator: Crown Corporations, Mac!

Mr. Chairman: I will brook no interruptions from the floor.

Mr. Douglas: Now, I know that this audience will give to Mr. Thatcher and myself a courteous hearing. I want to say that the reason for this debate is, that last year on the 22nd of May, in the course of the Pipeline Debate, Mr. Thatcher made a very strong attack on the Saskatchewan Crown Corporations. He made statements which in my opinion, were misleading and incorrect and consequently, I asked him to substantiate those statements in a public debate. I did so, not because I object to anyone criticizing the Crown Corporations. They are public enterprises and the business of public affairs. What I did object to was a member from Saskatchewan, standing up in the House of Commons, making statements which misrepresented his province. I have just returned from a series of meetings in Ontario. I found that at every meeting, Liberal candidates were getting on the platform and quoting the speech which Mr. Thatcher made and saying.

Mr. Chairman: I must inform the speaker he must not refer to the other speaker by name.

Mr. Douglas: I have known no rules of this procedure, Mr. Chairman. These rules were never read to me prior to this debate, but I will refer to him as the Liberal candidate, if that suits you better, Mr. Chairman.

Mr. Chairman: That is according to rules, Sir.

Mr. Douglas: And, I find that Liberal candidates across the country are quoting this speech, telling people that all the Crown Corporations in Saskatchewan have folded up, that they have been a dismal failure, and they say the best proof of it is that these statements were made by a man who lives in Saskatchewan and who is a former CCF Member of Parliament. I want to deal with that speech and I want to ask Mr. Thatcher, er... my opponent, when he is speaking to either substantiate the statements he made in the House of Commons or admit that he was misrepresenting the situation as far as these crown corporations are concerned.

Now, I can't quote all of his speech. That would take all of my 40 minutes. But, after all, you do not have to drink the whole pot of soup to know what the soup tastes like. All you need to have is a few spoonfuls. I am going to take some of the illustrations that were used by the Liberal candidate when he spoke in the House of Commons.

I will start with what he said about the Saskatchewan Housing Corporation. He said it has a deficit of $42,000. I have here the financial statement from which he must have been quoting. It is the only financial statement issued to the members of the legislature and to members of the Crown Corporations Committee. It has five columns: total net deficit, total net surplus, adjustments, net deficits, and net surpluses.

What does the Housing Corporation show? Housing Corporation shows, total net deficit of $42,000; an adjustment of $133,100; a net surplus of $90,700. What is the explanation for that? When we set up the Housing Corporation, we did so after the war to provide accommodation for veterans and their families. We provided some 445 suites. We provided accommodation and board for some 305 veterans and their families who were attending university. We did so under an agreement with the Central Mortgage and Housing Corporation by which they were to pay a certain amount in lieu of the contribution that would normally be coming from the federal government. We knew that money would come. It took some time in coming, but nevertheless it was part of the agreement. Therefore, we knew this $150,000 was coming and so there was not a deficit of $42,000; there is a surplus of $90,000. Why did my opponent quote the first column in the financial statement instead of the third column?

Now, my opponent is not an inexperienced boy. He is a university graduate in economics; he was for many years a high executive for Canada Packers; he has been a successful businessman; and for 12 years a member of the House of Commons. He knows what a financial report means and in the House of Commons he says that this crown corporation has a deficit of $42,000 when actually it had a surplus of $90,000. Moreover, he said that it closed up in 1947 leaving the impression that it went broke. It didn't close up. These houses are still being operated for veterans but they were turned over to the Department of Social Welfare, since the actual task of converting them into suites had been finished and it was a matter of continuing to operate.

This is the interesting thing. When this member was speaking about these buildings which turned into homes, he made no reference to the fact that the Saskatchewan Reconstruction Corporation, in turning war buildings and war assets into cash, had shown a return to the people of Saskatchewan of $395,000. When he was mentioning housing, why did he not mention the Reconstruction Corporation?

We'll take another example. My opponent referred to the Fish Marketing Service. He has spent much time castigating the Fish Marketing Board. Then he turned to the Fish Marketing Service and said 'although it has only been operating a few years, has accumulated a deficit of $180,000.' Now, this same financial statement which I have in my hand shows that it had that year a surplus—an operating surplus—of $30,417. Now, the only way I can account for this gentleman talking about an accumulated deficit of $180,000, is that he has taken into consideration the payments which were made by the Department of Natural Resources for floor prices for fishing.

Now, I know he does not believe in floor prices. In the House of Commons, he opposed the floor price of 58 cents a pound for butter and I have the Hansard here for anyone who wants to see it. He may not believe in floor prices, but the CCF government does believe in floor prices and over a period of years, we have paid out about $32,000 per year. Some years we didn't pay anything; some years we paid more. But the average was about $32,000 a year. We think that money was well spent. That money kept hundreds of fishermen from having to go on social aid; enabled them to earn a decent living, and gave them a guaranteed price for their catch.

Now, my opponent may not agree with floor prices, and that is his privilege. But the fact he doesn't agree with floor prices doesn't give him the right to take floor price payments made by the Department of Natural Resources and add it on to the operating expenses of the Marketing Board and call that a deficit, when actually there was an operating surplus of $30,417.

And to take another example. He made reference to the brick plant at Estevan. He said that the government sank $900,000 into this venture and had a deficit of $176,000. Now as a matter of fact, those figures are not quite right. The capital investment is $750,000. There was a write-off on the old plant of $102,000 making a total of $852,000, but my opponent took the $102,000 write-off and added it to the capitalization, and then he also added it to the accumulated deficit. Now, you can't count a write-off twice. If he does that with his income tax, he is going to get into trouble someday. You can't do that! So that at the time he was speaking, if you add the write-off to the capitalization, there was a capitalization of $852,000 and there was a deficit at the end of 1955 of $73,448 and the surplus for 1956 was wiped out. The deficit on the brick plant is now operating in the black.

Why didn't he tell the House of Commons all the facts? That this plant was started by a private company; that it closed in the 1930s, that it operated for only brief periods for the next 15 years; that the government re-opened it. Of course, we had difficulties with the operation because the equipment was old and obsolete. When we put in tunnel kilns, it immediately began to show good results.

Why didn't he tell the House of Commons, for instance, that if he were proud of Saskatchewan, that in 1953 the brick plant showed a surplus of $39,642 or 5.3% return on the capital investment; that in 1954, it showed a surplus of $36,672 or a 4.9% return on the capital investment; that in 1955, it showed a surplus of $56,986 or 7.6% return on the capital investment; and last year, it had a surplus of $70,000 and that the plant is now operating in the black.

Let me take a statement too, which my opponent made in reference to the sodium sulphate plant. He said several companies were operating in the province but the government, by passing legislation, forced these companies out of business or forced them to sell to the provincial government. Now, I submit, that statement is not correct. There were no regulations passed by the government to put any company out of business. What we did do is raise the royalty. The royalties were too low. Does my opponent object to the people of Saskatchewan getting a better return on their natural resources? And I want to remind you that the Crown Corporations pay the same royalties as we ask any private company to pay.

Now here is how we forced these people out of business: There are three sodium sulphate plants, privately owned, operating in the province now. One at Gladmar, in this constituency; one at Palo, and one at Ormeaux. Now it is true there was a plant at Bishopric started by a gentleman who was a friend of my opponent. He wanted to purchase a mine in South America, so he took out a mortgage on his Bishopric plant through an investment firm in New York. When he got into financial difficulties, the New York firm foreclosed on him. The New York firm did not want to operate the plant so they offered to the government and we purchased it. That plant is operating at Bishopric today; operating successfully, and giving a good return. So, we didn't put anybody out of business in sodium sulphate. We have a plant at Chaplin and a plant at Bishopric. Why didn't my friend, when he was making his speech about Crown Corporations, tell the House of Commons that in 1955 these sodium sulphate plants had accumulated profits of $659,000 and that they paid royalties of $287,000, making a total of $946,000. As a matter of fact, at the end of 1956, these two plants have paid in surpluses and royalties, $1,157,000 on a capital investment of only $1,085,000.

May I say something about the Saskatchewan Transportation Company? The member with whom I am debating tonight says that the investment in the Saskatchewan Transportation Company was $1,900,000 and was only able to make a nominal profit of $12,000. As a matter of fact, the capital investment is not $1,900,000 but $1,750,000 and when he talks about $12,000 he picks one year. He might just as well have picked 1949 when we had a surplus of $120,000. It would have been much fairer to have told the House of Commons that in the 11 years the Saskatchewan Transportation Company has been in operation, it has had an average profit of $33,000 a year; and at the end of 1955, it had an accumulated surplus of $370,000; at the end of 1956, it had an accumulated surplus of $432,000. And, in addition, my opponent didn't tell the House of Commons what he told the people of Moose Jaw, as reported in the Regina Leader Post on June 7, 1949 when he said this. I quote: "Mr. Thatcher says the bus company has opened up new lines and transportation facilities have been provided for people that were not existent previously."

Back in 1949, he recognized that the Saskatchewan Transportation Company was not just something to make money but something to open up areas which had no transportation facilities and thereby the government was giving a service, irrespective of the fact that the annual surplus was only nominal.

Now I probably come to the most amazing statement of all. My opponent then began to criticize the Government Insurance Office and he said that they secure business by compulsion. He said: "Everyone who wants to license his car or truck, must take insurance from the Saskatchewan Government Insurance Office."

Now, that statement is not true, just as everyone within the sound of my voice knows it is not true. Every dollar that is paid for insurance under the *Automobile Insurance Act* goes into the Automobile Insurance Fund. Not one dollar goes from that fund into the Saskatchewan Government Insurance Office. The only time that money goes out of that fund, it goes out to pay benefits to people who are injured or to the dependents of those who are killed. The Saskatchewan Government Insurance Office doesn't get a five-cent piece from the insurance on your car or your truck which you buy when you buy your license. Sure, if you buy a package policy, that is different. But on the compulsory insurance, the Saskatchewan Government Insurance Office doesn't get a nickel. Why does my opponent make a statement like that in the House of Commons where people can carry a story like that back to their communities?

The Automobile Accident Insurance Fund, at the end of 1955, had my opponent should have known this, a surplus of $2,694,000; at the end of 1956 it had a surplus of $3,404,000 which will not go into the Saskatchewan Government Insurance Office but which belongs to the automobile and truck drivers of Saskatchewan and will be used either to reduce rates or to increase the benefits of their insurance programme.

He then went on to say every hospital, sanitorium, school, orphanage, etc., must take out insurance with the S.G.I.O. Well, it is true, the government requires organizations to whom it paid heavy grants, both for construction and operation, to take out insurance with the Saskatchewan Government Insurance Office (S.G.I.O.) because if they should be so negligent so as not to have insurance, and their place burned down, we would be expected to put up very heavy commitments to build new schools or hospitals as the case might be. But why didn't my opponent tell the House of Commons that in 1954 this so-called compulsory insurance represented only 2% of the insurance we wrote, and in 1955 it represented less than 4.5% In other words, over 95% of the insurance done by the S.G.I.O. is done on a competitive basis with line insurance companies.

What is the result? The result is that at the end of 1955, the year under review, the Saskatchewan Government Insurance Office had an accumulated surplus of $2,291,000. And remember that not only do the people who buy insurance from the S.G.I.O. benefit, the rest of the people benefit. I have here photostatic copies of the rate book of the Canadian Insurance Underwriters Association, issued last June. What does it say? It says the prairie provinces ought to be divided into two zones. Zone I, Manitoba, Alberta, and Northwest Territories. Zone 2, Saskatchewan. Then it gives the rate for Zone 1. Then it says for Zone 2, deduct 20 percent. Everyone in the province who buys insurance is getting cheaper insurance by virtue of the fact that there is a Government Insurance Office.

Then my opponent proceeded to discuss three crown corporations which have closed up. The shoe factory, the tannery, and the woollen mill and said that these had cost the taxpayers of the province large sums of money.

Well, I want to point out in the first place we never suggested that every Crown Corporation that was set up would be an unqualified success. As President Roosevelt used to say, "You must trust us by our batting average. Sometimes we hit a home run, sometimes we strike out." But the Liberal Party makes a great deal of fuss about these three small crown corporations. What do they represent? They represent four-fifths of one percent of a total amount of money which the Saskatchewan people invested in crown corporations.

Now it is true that if these three corporations hadn't folded up, our surplus would have been bigger. That's true. But it is equally true that the people of Saskatchewan, as taxpayers, didn't pay anything. They got, as a matter of fact, a net surplus at the end of 1955 of $6,300,000 and at the end of 1956, a net surplus of $7,316,000. And if you add in power and telephone, at the end of 1955 we had a net surplus of $28.75 million and at the end of 1956, a net surplus of $34.4 million.

Now, my opponent got up in the House of Commons and told the people of Canada, and it was printed in almost every paper in this Dominion, that the Crown Corporations were a dismal failure. Well, let's look at the facts.

The people of this province invested in these Crown Corporations up to the end of 1955, $9,634,000, and in that year, they had a surplus after deducting losses of $1,366,000; or a return of 14.18 percent on the capital investment and in addition, they paid to the government royalties of $946,000.

Now, this is the point on which I would like to get some clarification from my opponent. Back in 1949, speaking in the city of Moose Jaw, as reported in the *Moose Jaw Times Herald*, my opponent said that "profits from the Crown Corporations had given a total overall investment return of 9 percent which is a pretty good return as any businessman may agree." Now what I want to know, if in 1949, 9 percent was a pretty good return, how come in 1956, 14 percent is a dismal failure?

And if we include power and telephones – we don't usually include then because our opponents say "well, of course, they're public monopolies" – but if you include power and telephones, then in 1955 the net surplus, after deducting losses, was $5,477,000 and in 1956, $5,717,000.

Now one of the things which surprised me about my opponent's speech in the House of Commons was that he found fault with the fact that Telephones were a government monopoly. Well, or course, any telephone company is a monopoly. Would my opponent prefer to have a private monopoly to a public monopoly? The Saskatchewan Telephone Corporation has served the people of this province well. When we took office in 1944, it had 47,000 customers; it now has over 135,000 customers. This public investment has gone from $16.5 million to $71 million.

Like the Power Corporation, when we took office in 1944, the Power Corporation had an accumulated deficit of $231,000. I want to point that out. That from the time the Power Corporation was established until 1946, the Power Corporation had an accumulated deficit every year. It wasn't until the CCF came into office in 1946, for the first time, we had a surplus and we now have in the Power Corporation an accumulated surplus of over $8.5 million.

But what is more important is the service which it has given. Since 1944, we have gone from 13,000 customers to 135,000 customers. We have gone from 137 farms with power to over 40,000 farms with power. We have gone from 146 communities with power to 793 communities with power. Our investment has gone up from $9 million to $148 million and natural gas, which we started in 1952, has gone from 300 customers to over 20,000 customers.

But the important thing is this: these are public utilities. They are public utilities in which there is no profit for a private investor. Every dollar of profit goes back to the people in reduced rates or in extended services.

Since 1949, there have been five reductions in power rates. Since we started gas, there already have been two reductions in the rates for natural gas.

Therefore, I ask any person to look at the overall picture which my opponent describes as a dismal failure.

I will say nothing about the indirect benefits of the Crown Corporations, although I could say much about that. Our Power Corporation alone uses one-quarter million tons of Saskatchewan coal each year and when their new plant is completed, they will be using one-half million tons. We have made business for the northern woodsman by using Saskatchewan coal. A company has come into the province to manufacture electric transformers; another company has come in to manufacture wire and cable because of our programme. We have a company now just getting ready to manufacture steel pipe because of our gas programme. Another company is going to manufacture multi-wall bags because of our sodium sulphate program in the province.

But, leaving out the indirect benefits, what have the people of Saskatchewan got out of these crown corporations in which their money has been invested?

Well, they have done in this past year a total of $56.5 million worth of business. It has given employment to over 4,500 persons with a payroll of $15.5 million. It shows a surplus, as I pointed out, in 1955, a net surplus after deducting losses of $5,477,000 and in 1956 of $5,717,000 and they have an accumulated surplus in 1955 of $28.75 million and last year of $34.4 million.

This is what my opponent describes to the people of Canada as a dismal failure. I say, that the Crown Corporations have done more to stimulate the economic life of this province and to give the people of this province service at cost, than anything else has ever done in the history of Saskatchewan.

Now as a matter of fact, I want to point out that the Crown Corporations haven't changed at all. It is my opponent who has changed! Back in 1949 he said, according to the *Moose Jaw Times Herald*, he said, "The provinces record on Crown Corporations is an indication of what would be achieved on a national scale by a CCF government."

And in the House of Commons, on June 5 1951, he said, "I am very proud of the CCF Party. I think they are doing an excellent job in Saskatchewan despite what is being said by the Liberal press. I like their hospitalization plan, their Crown Corporations, their financial achievements, their labour legislation, and just about everything else they have done."

And again, speaking in Moose Jaw on May 30 1952, he said, "The Crown Corporations have been a magnificent success while the housing situation in Canada is a national scandal."

I am, therefore, submitting that the Crown Corporations haven't changed at all. Crown corporations are in better financial shape today, are giving the people of this province better service today, than they were in 1949 and 1952, when my opponent made such complimentary remarks about them.

As a matter of fact, I submit, that the attack on the Saskatchewan Crown Corporations was made for only two reasons. The first is, that my opponent was going to vote against a CCF amendment to have the Trans-Canada Pipeline publicly owned. He had to have a reason for voting against it. He had just gone over to the other side. He had to prove to them that he was a genuine convert, that he really had got this public ownership bug out of his system, and, so therefore he had to get up to prove his good faith to his new party and make a vicious attack, and I say a complete series of false statements, against the Crown Corporations in his own native province.

The second reason he attacked the Crown Corporations was because he had to have some reason for deserting the people who in 1945, 1949, and 1953 had elected him to parliament with their money, their sweat, their toil, and votes. I am not criticizing any man for leaving a political party. Every man has a right to change his opinion. But, my opponent, prior to the 1953 election, when at his own nominating convention, they tackled him with the fact that he had opposed things which the CCF stood for, such as floor prices for farmers, higher family allowances, removing the means test on old age pensions...

Mr. Chairman: I must draw to the speaker's attention that he is straying a bit from the point.

Mr. Douglas: I am not straying, Mr. Chairman, I am going to make a point here.

I am pointing out that at that convention, my opponent stood up and said he would support the CCF programme; that he would support the principles of public ownership which, of course, would cover the Trans-Canada Pipeline and would cover the Crown Corporations we are talking about tonight.

I am told by Mr. M.J. Coldwell, who sat on the platform, that he said, "If the time comes when I cannot support this programme, I will come back and resign and let you people do what you will with me."

Now, I have no objection to a man changing his opinion. I have no objection to a man even leaving his Party, but I have objections to him breaking faith with his people who elected him and then maligning the Saskatchewan Crown Corporations, in an attempt to cover up his defection. As a matter of fact, this has to do with Crown Corporations too, one of the reasons he gave why he was leaving the CCF was he said there were too many Reds in the CCF.

Mr. Chairman: No more interruptions from the floor! This item is not, as far as I can see, anything to do with Crown Corporations, because they are not Red.

Mr. Douglas: I am now proposing to discuss whether or not they are Red and that's why they have to do with this matter.

My opponent has been going around this constituency, particularly in places which are not covered by the press, and he has been saying he knows things about people in the CCF and that he has photostatic copies of private file from the RCMP which show that there is a CCF MLA who has associations with the Communist party.

I am saying here, Mr. Speaker, that instead of discussing this in some private corner of the constituency, I am inviting the Liberal candidate to put this photostatic copy of the confidential file from the RCMP on this table. I am inviting him to tell me how he came into possession of a confidential file from the RCMP I want him to tell me whether or not he has that file with the knowledge and consent of Mr. Garson, the Minister of Justice, and to tell me whether or not Liberal candidates are being given confidential files from the police in order to carry out election campaigns.

And, I say, that this is part of the famous story of attacking crown corporations. Any kind of an excuse, whether saying that the CCF is too Red or whether it is saying that the crown corporations have been a dismal failure, saying that some of them have deficits, when as a matter of fact, they have surpluses, saying that the Saskatchewan Government Insurance Office takes the money when you buy your compulsory car insurance, when as a matter of fact we don't get any money at all. Statements like this, I maintain, were not made because the Saskatchewan Crown Corporations have not changed in any particular way. Saskatchewan Crown

Corporations are the same profit corporations which were operating when my opponent was a staunch supporter of the CCF movement. Crown Corporations haven't changed. They are doing better now than they did then. They are giving better service now. They are giving service to more people than they did then. I am saying the attack on the Saskatchewan Crown Corporations has done great harm to this province in other parts of Canada, was made to cover up the fact that my opponent has deserted and betrayed the people who elected him, and I say that any man who will use tactics like that in the House of Commons or anywhere else is not fit to represent the fine people of this constituency in the Parliament of Canada.

Mr. Chairman: The Liberal candidate for Assiniboia will now present his case and he will confine his remarks to the Crown Corporations of Saskatchewan. No interruptions from the floor please.

Mr. Thatcher: Mr. Chairman, Mr. Premier, Ladies and Gentleman.

First of all, it is a pleasure for me to be here tonight in the town of Mossbank, particularly for the purpose of debating Saskatchewan's Crown Corporations.

I felt a moment ago that perhaps the Premier was a little bitter. I can't say that I blame him for not talking about Crown Corporations at all for the last ten minutes of his speech because the record is pretty bad. The Premier said that my speech has done great disservice to my province in the east. I believe it has done great disservice to the CCF Party and I hope that that is true.

Now, Mr. Chairman, how did this debate come about? In May 1956, as the Premier told you, I made a speech in the House of Commons pertaining to the record of Saskatchewan's Crown Corporations. Five months later, the Premier, at the Assiniboia CCF Nominating Convention took violent exception to my remarks.

Well, now in the first place, he charged that I lacked courage to make those statements in Saskatchewan where I could be answered. Very respectfully, I will tell the Premier that I have made those speeches on many platforms in Saskatchewan, but even if this were not so, I fail to see how the Premier can object to a Member of Parliament speaking on any subject in the House of Commons. When I made that speech to which my opponent objects, CCF federal members, including, I believe, my opponent in the Assiniboia constituency, were there. They had every opportunity, in debate, to refute either the statements made or the figures used.

Now, according to newspaper reports of that Assiniboia nominating convention, the Premier challenged me to debate the subject on any public platform. He said in effect, "He may as well make up his mind to have a joint meeting, because I shall hound him from one end of the constituency to the other." Well, Mr. Chairman, I know that the Premier is a busy man and I wouldn't want him spending all his time down in this constituency, although he has been spending a good deal. Therefore, I am happy to accept his challenge.

Well, Mr. Chairman, the original Crown Corporation programme was launched shortly after the CCF came to power in 1944. Prior to that date, Socialist speakers constantly deprecated the fact that private enterprise had not established industry in Saskatchewan and they deplored the fact, and rightly I think, that thousands of young citizens in Saskatchewan in those days were forced to go down to the United States or to B.C. or down east to find employment. One of the CCF planks which appealed to me most, as a young man, was the promise to end this situation.

Now the Premier, and all Socialists from the Premier down, said, "If private capital would not establish industry in Saskatchewan, we shall do it ourselves by state ownership and thus provide employment." And at the same time, the Premier and CCF spokesman promised the people extensive, free social services and these services were to be financed in considerable part from the profits of government-owned industries. I quote the *Regina Leader Post* of June 13, 1944 where the Premier said, "The CCF proposes to get money for its social service program by the government engaging in revenue producing businesses."

Now, these then I say respectfully, Mr. Chairman, were the original objectives in this experiment in state socialism. I frankly admit that no one supported that programme more enthusiastically than I. That is, until I learned the true facts.

Since taking office, the Socialist government has either set up or taken over 19 Crown Corporations. And in those companies, as nearly as I can ascertain at the present time, they have invested approximately $175 million of taxpayer's money. After 12 years of experimentation, I suggest that three questions be posed and considered by the people of Saskatchewan tonight.

First of all, have the Crown Corporations been able to operate efficiently?

Secondly, has the government, because of the programme, been able to provide a substantial number of additional jobs for Saskatchewan citizens in manufacturing industries?

Thirdly, have the Crown Corporations made revenue available to the provincial treasury which it could use for social services, highways, school grants etc?

I believe the answers to these three questions will tell us whether state socialism in Saskatchewan has succeeded or failed.

Well now, let us look for a moment at some of the individual companies. One of the first enterprises set up was the leather tannery. What are the facts pertaining to that company? The purpose of the leather tannery was to tan cowhides and make them into leather. 1946 was a year of short supplies and high prices, the best possible condition under which to commence operating an industry. And yet the activities of the tannery were ill-fated and short lived. About the only hides they tanned were the hides of the Saskatchewan taxpayers.

And so, the company moved from one economic crisis to another until December, 1948, when the employees were thrown out of work just before Christmas. And when all the smoke had cleared away, that company has a deficit, as nearly as I can ascertain, of roughly $200,000. One company up, one company down!

A shoe factory was set up in 1945 to utilize the leather which was made in the tannery. What are the facts pertaining to the shoe factory? I recall Premier Douglas speaking at Brandon, Manitoba, and he announced and I quote from his speech: "The tannery and shoe factory now being operated by the CCF can make shoes for $2.75 a pair". Well, in spite of the Premier's optimism on that occasion, the shoe factory did lose money, so much so that in 1948, it closed down after having accumulated deficits of more than $82,000. Two companies up, two companies down!

A woollen mill was set up in my home city of Moose Jaw. What are the facts pertaining to that this operation? The paper theory behind this operation was reasonable, but the industry was in difficulty from its opening day. When it was finally forced to close in 1951, it had accumulated deficits of $830,000 and it paid none of the interest on its $206,000 of advances. The mill was transferred to a private company. That company finally moved the machinery out of the province and today the whole operation is defunct. Three companies up, three companies down!

And now I come to the Housing Corporation. The Housing Corporation was set up after the war to convert military huts into housing accommodation that could be rented. And it should be noted that the CCF government, which has been so noisy in its demands for the federal government to build low rent housing, has done virtually nothing in this field itself. We have one of those housing projects in the City of Moose Jaw up near the Exhibition Grounds. I have seen better housing condemned for slum clearance.

And yet despite the fact that CCF progress in building housing was extremely limited, in a relatively short period of time, the Housing Corporation was able to accumulate deficits of $42,000. Now, the Premier said tonight my figures are wrong. "Why," he said, "there should have been a federal government grant in that figure." Well, I have a question in my hand which was asked of Mr. Fines on February 21, 1956. That question was this: *What audited statement of report shows an accumulated surplus of $90,699 for Saskatchewan Reconstruction Housing Corporation?* His answer was, *"No audited statement or report shows an accumulated surplus of $90,699 for the Saskatchewan Reconstruction Housing Corporation."*

Now, the government, as it time and time again does, takes a federal grant or a provincial grant and suddenly puts it in the revenue account of a Crown Corporation and then turns around and says that actually it has been making money. That Housing Corporation in 1947 was closed down despite what the Premier says. That is four companies up, four companies down!

Very early in its first term of office, the CCF government set up a Fish Board, and they built a number of fish filleting plants in northern Saskatchewan. Every commercial fisherman in a defined area was compelled to sell his fish to the Board. Despite that fact, almost from its inception the Corporation lost money and I think the situation was all the worse because it frequently paid the fisherman less than they could have obtained from private buyers. After accumulating a deficit of roughly $400,000, which as usual did not contain interest on advances, the government closed it down in 1949. Five companies up, five companies down!

The Fish Board was then replaced by the Fish Marketing Service. From the start, the government concealed the losses of this new Board by making an annual grant and at the end of the last fiscal year, the Premier told us they were showing a surplus of $32,000. In fact, I say that figure is a little more than fiction because to arrive at this amount, provincial grants of $242,000 are included as revenue.

In 1951, the lumber mill was set up at Big River, Saskatchewan. Within a year and a half, the mill reported a deficit of more than $97,000 and it cost the treasury another $54,000 in interest on advances. Well, having thus demonstrated itself subject to heavy deficits in 1953 it was merged with the Timber Board. Since then, its results have been concealed under the surpluses or behind the surpluses of the Timber Board.

The box factory at Prince Albert was expropriated from a private corporation under pretty drastic legislation. The manager of the plant, when it was under private ownership, was ordered by some of the government socialist planners to follow a certain course of action. He refused on the grounds that such a policy would bankrupt him. The Socialists then moved in and confiscated the plant. Since that day, the box factory has been in financial difficulty. During the last year alone, according to the government's own figures, it had a loss of $133,000, bringing its accumulated deficits to the rather shocking total of $352,000. That whole operation has been a fiasco, and should be sold back to a private company that knows the economic facts of life.

A broken-down brick plant in Estevan was purchased by the government shortly after the war, and since that time approximately $750,000 in capital investment has been put by the government into this venture. Now, despite the fact that most government agencies and most government departments, when putting up new buildings, have been ordered to use brick from this plant; despite the fact that Canada since 1945 has enjoyed the greatest construction boom in her history; from its inception, this brick plant has experienced engineering difficulties, technical difficulties, selling difficulties, over-production and high employee layoff.

According to the government's own figures, up to March 1956, the company had a deficit of $105,000. The Premier tells us tonight that this has now been wiped out, but if interest on advances is included, and why shouldn't it be, the true picture shows the deficit would be very substantial even today.

Now, Mr. Chairman, in the cases I have mentioned so far there was competition from private enterprise. I think it is significant to know that under these circumstances, in virtually every case, the Crown Corporation was unable to compete effectively. Invariably they lost money, and usually they were forced to close their doors completely.

What of the other Crown Corporations? The Premier tonight has boasted that some of them have shown substantial profits. In some cases, this has been true, but almost without exception, closer examination and analysis show the only companies which have made money are those which have enjoyed government compulsion, some form of monopoly, some special government privilege.

The Saskatchewan Government Printing Company is a good example. Over the years it has accumulated net profits of slightly more than $500,000. Why shouldn't it? The printing company is supplied by the government with all the work it can do, from the most profitable printing jobs and at non-competitive prices.

The Telephone Company has been one of the major money makers. And it should be remembered that the Telephone Company was originally set up by the Liberals in 1908 and this is a company which we do believe lends itself to social ownership. Of course, it enjoys a virtual monopoly in the province over telephones, with the exception of a few rural lines.

The Premier told us tonight that one of the big advantages of public ownership is that it can serve people even where it is not profitable. Well, there are many farmers in this province who wonder why this Socialist government, whose slogan is "humanity first has steadily refused to take over some of the unprofitable rural lines in many areas of the province.

The Timber Board is one of the most profitable of all these Crown Corporations and up to the end of last year it accumulated surpluses of $3.5 million. How did it do so? The Socialist government gave the Timber Board an almost complete monopoly of lumber harvested in Saskatchewan. Producers are compelled by law to sell their timber to this Board at relatively low prices. Then the Board goes out into the high markets of Canada and the United States and resells the lumber. The company does provide employment for many people. Yet, it is also a fact that its operations have resulted in the closing down of many private sawmills and associated businesses.

The government some years ago established a Fur Marketing Board and that company has an operating surplus. Once again, the reason for this rather unique situation is not hard to find. All trappers were originally forced by law to sell their beaver and muskrat skins through the board. Speaking over the radio on April 3, 1957, our provincial network, the Honorable A.J. Kuziak, Minister of Natural Resources boasted that "the elimination of the middleman between the manufacturer and the trapper has put money into the pockets of our trappers and has meant a higher standard of living." Well, Mr. Chairman, apparently the trapper did not appreciate these socialist benefits because they strongly agitated for and voted for a discontinuance of this state monopoly. Such was the dissatisfaction among trappers that the government was forced during the 1955-56 season to permit open markets. Profits, as a result, have dropped sharply in the past year.

Now I come to the Saskatchewan Government Insurance Office. The Saskatchewan Government Insurance Office has had substantial financial growth as the Premier has pointed out. Speaking on the provincial radio network again, Mr. Kuziak had this to say; he claimed that the company was commenced in 1945 with a government investment of $12,000.

"Today," he boasted, "it has assets of over $12 million" and that is half a truth. Mr. Kuziak deliberately neglected to mention that the company also had liabilities of $9,600,000. The Insurance Company, since its inception in 1945, has accumulated a surplus of $2,340,000. At first glance this surplus is very gratifying. I want tonight to apologize to the Premier that auto insurance went into this fund. That was my original belief. I was in error, sir, and I apologize for it.

However, when you examine the facts, you still find that a good deal of the business of the Insurance Company has been obtained by compulsion. For example, all institutions, as the Premier mentioned, such as schools, hospitals, health units, orphanages, sanitaria, and the like receiving government grants must purchase their insurance from the Saskatchewan Government Insurance Office. And I would like to point out moreover that many government buildings that were formerly not insured by previous administrations because they were fireproof, today take out insurance with the government. Now, all this business is obtained at non-competitive rates and with no solicitation costs.

The Premier claims that the Saskatchewan Government Insurance Office forced all other companies in Saskatchewan to reduce rates in Saskatchewan, and at one time I think that was the case, but today the opposite is frequently true. Both board and non-board companies are frequently underselling the government company. Repeatedly these private companies are forcing the Government Insurance Office to reduce rates in order to compete. As a result of private competition in this last year, the Government Insurance Company had an underwriting loss of $132,000. The Saskatchewan Guarantee and Fidelity Company was purchased by the government in 1949 at a cost of $250,000 and this company since its inception has accumulated surpluses but once again a considerable portion of the business has been obtained by compulsory methods. For example, owners of commercial trucks and of public service vehicles are compelled by law to purchase various kinds of insurance and guarantee bonds from this company. Electrical contractors, gas contractors, electrical supply houses, are likewise ordered to buy guarantee bonds from this company. On the type of business where it has to compete, the company has steadily run into increasing difficulties. So much so that in the last fiscal year the Saskatchewan Guarantee and Fidelity Company had a net loss of $103,000.

The Saskatchewan Transportation Company was set up after the CCF took over. It took upon itself a monopoly of those bus routes which were not inter-provincial by their nature. A number of private operators had their bus lines arbitrarily expropriated. For example, we have one man in this audience tonight who had his bus business confiscated by the government. He is Mr. H.B. Legge of Moose Jaw who had operated a bus line from Moose Jaw to Riverhurst for seven years. Overnight he was put out of business to make way for the government company. Now the ironic feature of the Legge case is the fact that the government after operating the line for a short period of time, finding it unprofitable, abandoned it. CCF speakers claim that the Saskatchewan Transportation Company provides service to areas where private enterprise won't go. Well, the Moose Jaw-Riverhurst line would indicate that in some instances citizens were deprived of a service they previously enjoyed under private enterprise.

Despite the monopolistic character of this operation, the Saskatchewan Transportation Company has shown only nominal profits, six-tenths of one percent on its investment in 1955 and 3.5 percent in 1956. Had it paid interest on its advances, it actually would have lost substantial sums of money.

The Saskatchewan Power Corporation was set up by the Liberal government in 1928. Power is a field which we also admit lends itself to social ownership. Yet I also believe that under the CCF government, the results have been anything but efficient. The Power Corporation has worked gradually towards a monopoly in the distribution of electricity. It has established a complete monopoly in the distribution of gas. Now, let us look first at the field of electricity.

I believe in giving credit where credit is due and I freely admit that the Power Corporation since 1945 has done a good job of bringing electricity to rural areas. But it has done no better job than a Liberal government in Manitoba of a Social Credit government in Alberta.

Ladies and gentlemen, I believe it is a fair statement to say that we would have had rural electrification in Saskatchewan since 1945 regardless of what party had been in power. Today, there are farmers in our province who have great difficulty finding the $550 down payment to put electricity into their yards. In Manitoba, electricity is brought to a farm with no initial down payment, since the original cost is amortized over a period of years and included in the monthly light bill. And I admit very frankly that to get that sort of a deal you have to buy some appliances, but I still say that it is a better deal than the farmer gets in Saskatchewan.

Now ladies and gentlemen, you heard the Leader of the Socialist Party in Saskatchewan tonight refer with pride to the fact that in the past few years the Power Corporation has been able to put five different rate reductions into effect. Well, if that is so, I say those rates are still very high, still very far out of line and still very excessive. For example, under a Liberal administration in Manitoba, power rates to farmers are substantially less than they are in Saskatchewan. For 200 kilowatt hours, a Manitoba farmer pays $5.85; $9.99 in Saskatchewan; for 300 kilowatt hours, a Manitoba farmer pays $6.75; $11.38 in Saskatchewan; for 400 kilowatt hours, 7.65 in Manitoba, $12.93 in Saskatchewan. In other words, the Saskatchewan rate are roughly 70 percent higher than comparable Manitoba rates, after the five reductions the Premier mentioned.

Now, here in Saskatchewan, we are fortunate I think to have one private utility left in the province, the National Light and Power Company. This company serves the City of Moose Jaw, but it also serves a number of rural lines. The comparison of the rates between the private utility and the crown corporation shows a glaring difference. For example, I have with me tonight, the rate schedule of the Saskatchewan Power Corporation and the National Light and Power Company. A farmer on a National Light and Power line using 500 kilowatt hours pays $9.25 per month. The farmer on the government line pays $14.05, approximately 52 percent higher, and that prevails across the board. Now about three years ago, there were 50 farmers in the Crestwynd area who asked the Power Corporation to supply them with power. They were informed that some years might elapse before their request could be granted. The farmers than asked if the National Light and Power Company could be given a permit to service them immediately. The permit was granted, but only on condition that National Light and Power charge the Power Corporation rates. In other words, here we have a government that professes to believe in "humanity first" forcing 50 farmers in the Crestwynd area to pay between 50 and 60 percent more for their electricity than the private company wants to charge them. Why? Simply to hide from the people in that area the huge difference which exists between National Light rates and government rates. And, I may say, ladies and gentlemen, that the city of Prince Albert, which is served by the Power Corporation– in most cases pays up to 30 percent more for their electricity than the citizens of Moose Jaw under the National Light and Power Company.

Now, let us look at the field of gas. The Power Corporation, of course, have set up a gas monopoly. The Premier has made this statement on a number of occasions, and I think he made it tonight. "The great advantage of public utilities is that they operate on a service-at-cost basis." Well, as far as gas is concerned, I say that this is quite an admission for the Premier to make because it certainly follows that Power Corporation gas costs are far, far out of line when compared to Alberta companies, whether public or private.

Now, I have with me tonight the rate charges for gas in three Alberta cities: Medicine Hat, Calgary, and Edmonton. And I also have the Power Corporation charges. The difference, to say the least, is shocking. 30,000 cubic feet of gas is normal consumption for a Canadian home in winter. The rate for this amount of gas in Medicine Hat is $8.10; in Edmonton

$9.15; in Calgary $9.78, in Moose Jaw $19.26. In other words, ladies and gentlemen the government monopoly in the gas field in Saskatchewan is charging double, or 2.5 times as much as public or private enterprise is charging in the province of Alberta. Is that socialist efficiency?

Now, I remind the Premier further that the Trans-Canada Pipeline, which his party maligned for days in the House of Commons this past session, offered to deliver gas to the City of Moose Jaw for 21.3 cents, the cost of distribution over and above that, of course, would be another 15 cents. But that 36 cent total is a far cry from the 68 to 70 cents being charged by our Socialist government today to Saskatchewan consumers. Small wonder that the Saskatchewan Power Corporation can afford to spend such large sums of money for propaganda on television, on radio, and in newspapers. And, I say flatly that the Power Corporation rates which are being charged to the people of Saskatchewan are little short of a provincial scandal.

Now, I return, Mr. Chairman to the first question which I posed earlier. Have the Crown Corporations been able to operate efficiently? An interested observer finds it an almost unbelievable task to learn the true facts because time and again in the Crown Corporations Committee of the legislature, opposition members have been refused information on the grounds that it would not be in the public interest. Moreover, every possible accounting device, no matter how unorthodox, has been used to maintain the fiction that the industries are profitable and that socialism has been successful.

What are some of the devices used to hide the true facts? Time will only permit me to mention a few. In the first place, no interest is paid on advances made by the treasury, except in the case of the Power and Telephone companies. Can you imagine a private company not listing interest on borrowed money as an expense? Frequently, direct provincial grants to a corporation are carried in the profit and loss statement as revenue. In order to organize and operate the industry, the CCF government appointed an

Economic Advisory and Planning Board. Salaries to that Board amount to $50,000 per year, yet they are not charged to the Crown Corporations; they are paid out of the general finds of the province. And the auditing expenses of all these corporations are similarly treated. They are not paid by the Crown Corporations. They are paid directly by the taxpayers of the province, and the total of those auditing expenses since the government started its Crown Corporations is $449,000. In other instances, the cost of the Corporations has been paid by departments of government.

Well now, Mr. Chairman, the Premier told us tonight these companies had made 14.18 percent on their investment. When he made that percentage statement he simply ignored all the charges I have just mentioned. In order to arrive at that figure, he has indulged in a fantastic example of arithmetical gymnastics.

First of all, he threw out altogether from his calculation the telephone and power corporations. Apparently, their percentage return was too low. Then in computing the profits of the other companies, he overlooked interest on advances, he overlooked auditing expenses, he overlooked the salaries of the Planning Board, he overlooked loss on disposal of assets. Mr. Chairman, on page 11 of his Budget Speech, Mr. Fines claims profits of the Telephone and Power companies were $4,700,000 and he also claimed the total investment of the taxpayers to date is $162 million. On page three of the government finance office report, profits of the other companies are claimed to be $1,233,000. Now, according to the Crown Corporation auditors themselves, all the companies last year made not 14.18 percent, they made 3.7 percent. And if all expenses had been properly charged, they would have made 3.4 percent.

Now, what about the up-to-date financial picture? The Premier told us that up to date all these Crown Corporations with the exception of the Power and the Telephone companies have a surplus of $6,372,000. Well, I know the Premier is not a businessman, but I believe he should realize that he overlooked many debits which should have been applied against this figure. And I mention only a few:

$2,289,000 in interest on investment, which the people had to pay!

$498,000 in grants, which the people had to pay!

$565,000, the cost of operating the Finance Office, which the people had to pay!

$307,000 for the government purchase of assets of defunct corporations, which the people had to pay!

$449,000 for auditing expenses, which the people had to pay!

And there are other expenses which should be included. Now, these figures drop the real surplus from the $6,372,000 that the Premier mentioned to $2,264,000. A far cry, I may say, from the approximately $50 million that the Premier and Mr. Fines have claimed over the years that these companies have made.

Now in analyzing these overall results, we should bear in mind that none of these companies has paid any federal corporation taxes. Of course, most of them made enough money anyway, so I don't suppose this is a serious item. But, for most of their lives, they have also paid no municipal taxes.

Now, for all these reasons, Mr. Chairman, despite the extravagant claims made by the Leader of the Socialist Party of Saskatchewan tonight, I can only conclude that these industries have failed to produce any genuine or substantial profits with the exception of the three major monopolies.

A number of the companies, which in 1945, the Premier told us heralded a new economic and social order, have gone broke. Other companies which have had to compete with privately owned industry have almost invariably lost money. Practically without exception the only companies which have been able to show substantial profits have been those with a monopoly or special government privilege. Even this latter class has displayed very little efficiency. The excessive rates charged by the corporation for electricity and gas are typical.

Well now that the failure of many of these socialist ventures is well demonstrated, the Premier has tried tonight to create the impression that they were not expected to provide profits, but were organized for some other purpose. Well, he did not talk thus in 1944.

The second objective of the programme was to provide better employment opportunities in manufacturing industries for our young people in Saskatchewan. I remind you that since the war, manufacturing capacity in Canada has tripled. Thousands of new plants have been built, thousands of plants have been extended, hundreds of thousands of new workers have been employed.

Now, what about manufacturing in Saskatchewan? On April 17, 1957, Mr. Chairman, I wrote the Dominion Bureau of Statistics and I asked them a very simple question: *how many people were engaged in Saskatchewan in manufacturing industries in 1945 and how many were engaged in 1956?* And, Mr. Chairman, I shall table these figures for your perusal as soon as I finish speaking. They are indeed shocking, because they show that despite the spending of $175 million by the CCF government in Crown Corporations, despite the fact that manufacturing everywhere else in Canada has doubled or tripled, we have at the end of last year 67 less people in manufacturing than in the first year of the CCF being in office. In other words, I say that these corporations have failed in their second major objective and I challenge the Premier to show that this is not so in his rebuttal.

Now, the third purpose of the Crown Corporation programme, as I mentioned earlier, was to provide money for social services, highways, education etc. Has the programme succeeded in this regard? Well, quoting from the Premier's radio speech of October 24, 1956, he said that the Saskatchewan Government has never received a five-cent piece from power, gas, or telephone operation.

I will go further, Mr. Chairman, than the Premier did. I will say flatly that the companies have never paid a five-cent piece to social services, roads, highways, or schools, or anything of the kind. As a matter of fact, ladies and gentlemen, quite the contrary is true. Millions have been drained off by this Socialist government, spent in costly Socialist experiments. This money would otherwise would have been available for better old age pensions, better educational and municipal grants, better highways etc...

The Leader of the Socialist Party tells us that the Crown Corporations have done more than any single thing to stimulate Saskatchewan's industrial development. In my opinion, such a statement is nonsense. Instead, the Crown Corporations are one of the reasons why Saskatchewan has lagged so far behind our other provinces in industrial growth. The threat of expropriation, the competition from government-owned industries paying no taxes, and the impractical theories of socialist planners, have discouraged private investors from coming into Saskatchewan in a fantastic manner and have retarded industrial development.

I have in my hand a letter from one of the largest gold mining companies on the North American Continent. This particular company was interested in investing in a sodium sulphate plant in Saskatchewan back in 1949 and I am going to table the letter with the Chairman. This gentleman wrote as follows:

"After due consideration of the market possibilities, and a rather detailed consideration of the political aspects of the Saskatchewan provincial government, I have regretfully come to the conclusion that as long as the provincial government's attitude is as it is today, there do not exist in the development of Ingebright Lake economic possibilities to justify our participation in such a

venture. Given free enterprise, under a reasonably Conservative government, I believe that Ingebright could not only hold its own but oust several of the existing producers on the basis of profit."

Now, that letter, ladies and gentlemen is typical of the companies that have been kept out of this province by the Socialist theory of the present government in Regina. Today, when the Premier talks about industrial development in our province he refers only to the results of the investments of the capitalists, who in 1944 he depicted as our chief public enemies. Any Saskatchewan development that we have had in the last ten years has been largely due to private enterprise such as oil and uranium and the like.

The Premier says, "But the Liberals have Crown Corporations." He says, "The Liberal corporations are operated themselves." Well, that is true, but Mr. C.D. Howe made a rather profound statement, the other night in Weyburn. He said, "The federal companies, almost without exception, are making substantial sums of money under proper management."

Well, I would say this: most of the federal companies which are socially owned were born either in the emergency of war or for some special reason when private enterprise could not do the job required. The Liberals believe in state ownership, but only as a last resort.

Now, these are the facts, Mr. Chairman. These are the facts that prompted me to say last May 22nd that the Crown Corporation programme has bogged down in a morass of bungling, red tape, and inefficiency, and after 12 years the programme has failed to achieve any of its major objectives. Even the Premier must apparently have realized this fact, because I believe it is eight years now since any new experiment has been launched. The CCF government, in 12 years of being in office, has rapidly demonstrated through its crown corporation programme, the futility of Socialism but at a terrible cost to the Saskatchewan taxpayer.

Mr. Chairman, I have presented my case to prove that the Saskatchewan

Crown Corporations programme has been a costly failure. It has failed in every respect to accomplish its original objective.

In the first place, despite the claims of the Premier, these industries have failed to produce any substantial overall profits, with the exception of the Power and Telephone companies, started by the Liberals, and the Timber Board, which the government runs as a rigid state monopoly.

In the second place, Mr. Chairman, despite a huge investment of the taxpayer's money, the companies have failed to increase the total overall industrial jobs available in Saskatchewan.

In the third place, despite original hopes, the corporations have failed to produce a single dollar which has been used to provide better social services, better educational grants, better highways, etc., for the people of Saskatchewan. In fact, the contrary is true.

And, in the fourth place, I would say that the programme has discouraged industrialists from investing in Saskatchewan and, largely as a result of this fact, our province lags behind our sister provinces in manufacturing development.

Now, the Leader of the Socialist Party has made his case. He can neither add to it nor subtract from it in the time remaining for his rebuttal. He may only refer to the points I have made in argument and bring evidence to show my facts are in error.

Ladies and gentlemen, you have heard the Premier speak to you for 40 minutes. During that time, he has failed to do two things: he has failed to prove that the Crown Corporation programme has achieved its original objectives. Second, he has failed to refute my basic contentions. Why has he failed? Because he cannot refute them! Facts are facts and I submit, ladies and gentlemen, that up to now the Premier has failed to establish a case for Saskatchewan's Crown Corporations. Socialism in Saskatchewan, as far as the Crown Corporations are concerned, has been tried and found wanting.

Now, ladies and gentlemen, I could say a few bitter things about the Premier, just as he will likely do in the next 10 minutes about me. However, I have tried to stick to facts. That is my case, and I think the facts are not refutable.

Thank You, Mr. Chairman.

Mr. Chairman: The meeting will come to order please. The Premier of Saskatchewan has now 10 minutes for rebuttal and I ask you to give him your attention.

Mr. Douglas: Ladies and gentlemen, I have only 10 minutes and, therefore, I will not waste any of it in preliminaries.

My opponent who just sat down told you that he was interested and believed that there were two things that ought to be publicly owned. The one was Power and the other was Telephones and he said that Mr. C.D. Howe, the other evening in Weyburn, made a profound statement that the 29 federal Crown Corporations were making money. In the light of that, I am interested in the statement which Mr. Thatcher made while speaking on November 9, 1955 in Toronto, to the Canadian Tax Foundation Conference, when he said, "I am rather of the opinion that the day has come when the federal government should consider selling such companies as Trans-Canada Airlines, Polimar Corporation, and others to private industry at a fair price. I m sure the taxpayer would benefit."

Whether they make money or not, my opponent is in favor of turning them over to private enterprise, So, apparently, he doesn't even agree with the Liberal government's policy of Crown Corporations. I say to my Liberal friends here, we had him yesterday, you have him today, heaven only knows who will have him tomorrow.

I am going to deal with the three main headings, and since I only have a few minutes, I can only touch a minute or two on each. My opponent dealt with three points: Were the Crown Corporations efficient? Did they create employment? Did they give revenues? I will deal with these points one by one.

One, are they efficient? He tried to prove they were not efficient by quoting rates. For instance, he talked about power being cheaper in Manitoba than in Saskatchewan. Of course, it is. In Manitoba the government started to put in rural power 30 years ago. We had a Liberal government in Saskatchewan that did nothing about putting in power. We put in power when materials were costing four and five times what it cost in Manitoba, plus the fact, of course, that we had to travel many more miles to supply the same number of customers as they do in Manitoba. He compared gas rates. He was very careful to compare gas rates with Medicine Hat, Calgary, and Edmonton who put in their gas systems 30 years ago when steel cost a fifth of the cost per ton that it is today. Those firms have already paid off their capital investment and today are charging only operating costs plus a good profit.

Why doesn't he make a comparison, however, with the Saskatchewan rates with something that is being built today. What do we find? We find for instance that gas in the City of Winnipeg for heating only is going to cost $1.14 as compared to 76.4 cents in Regina and for heating and cooking $1.12 compared to 72 cents. Now, of course there is a difference in the distance. But the difference in the distance [that the gas has to be piped], and depending on the load factor, (assume there is a 40 percent load factor), is a difference of 11.75 cents and it is 100 percent from a difference of 3.46 cents. Therefore, even taking out the difference [in distance] of the two areas of some 400 miles, which costs on the average, assuming an average load factor, about 6 cents, the difference is between 31 and 34 cents for 1000 cubic feet that the people of Winnipeg are paying more for their gas than the citizens of Regina or Moose Jaw who are getting it under a publicly owned enterprise.

Now, he says, that insurance companies are forcing Saskatchewan Government Insurance to raise rates. Well, I have got the rates here, for instance for the little town of Mossbank. If you take the board and independent companies, their rates for class one and two package [policies], groups 55 and 59 as compared to our 45, their class one and two underproved groups 60 and 55, compared to our 50 and 50. I won't bother reading them out. I have the same rates for Assiniboia, Gravelbourg, Estevan, and Weyburn. I will leave it with the Chairman to say that every one of these rates for the Saskatchewan Government Insurance Office is less than the comparable rates for the Board companies and for Wawanesa.

My friend wants to compare rates by taking the few farmers who are supplied by National Light and Power from Moose Jaw. It supplies 232 farmers as compared with eight or nine thousand urban customers. Saskatchewan Power Corporation, remember, doesn't supply power to the citizens of Regina, Moose Jaw, Saskatoon, or Weyburn. The result is that whereas National Light and Power has 35 urban customers for every rural customer; we have 2.2 urban customers for every rural customer and we also cover a much larger area. As a matter of fact, if private companies can supply power cheaper, why didn't the private companies that were here before we bought them out put up rural electrification?

Why, in 1944, there were only 137 farms with power. My opponent says "Ah, but Alberta, look what they have done." They have made the farmer pay the whole cost of the line. The farmers in Alberta are paying from $1,200 to $1,800 to get the power line in and then they have to maintain the power and replace the power line when it is worn out.

Spectator: Then they own it!

Mr. Douglas: Yes, they own it!

Now, my opponent has next raised the question of employment. He said he challenged me to show that there is more employment now than in

1944. And he is taking the figures with which I am quite familiar, from the federal Department of Labour, which only considers firms' statistics or from the Dominion Bureau who get them from the Department of Labour–and they only take figures in a plant which, unless it is above a certain size, otherwise they don't count the figures at all.

The figures we have for all employment…

Well, my friends may groan, but the fact is that is how the figures are computed, unless….

As a matter of fact, these statistics cover only manufacturing, and total numbers of people industrially employed, there are 10,000 more jobs in Saskatchewan today than there was in 1944. And as compared with 1941, when only 30 percent of the people lived in urban communities, today 50.2 live in urban communities. My opponent says that industry has been frightened away from the province because of the Crown Corporations. Well, if you look at the public and private investment figures for the last year, what do you find? You find that across Canada public and private investment went up 6 percent but in Saskatchewan it went up by 10 percent; higher than the national average. Public and private investment in Saskatchewan last year was $17 million higher than in the Province of Manitoba. Why doesn't the Liberal Party tell you those kinds of facts? As a matter of fact, the Liberal Party would rather malign this province and see it a desolate waste, than see it succeed under a CCF government.

Now, the last point of my opponent is the most amazing of all. He says of revenue, "I am prepared to say that not a five-cent piece has ever gone from the Crown Corporations into the provincial treasury." I wonder where he got that information, but if he will take the trouble to look over the receipts and expenditures of the provincial government, he will find that every year since 1955, there is no year that less than $0.5 million has been paid by the Government Finance Office into the provincial treasury. Not a single year!

Now, since 1945—now this is the kind of thing these people like to go round the country making sweeping statements about—not a single five cent piece, not a single five cent piece.

As a matter of fact, the Crown Corporations have not only paid money into the provincial treasury but every dollar in addition has been plowed back into the extension of services. Of the $34.4 million surplus at the end of 1956, that has been plowed back into providing more power, more services, more gas, for the people of the province. And I want to say this, that I believe the people of this province recognize that the Crown Corporations have made a genuine contribution to the economic life of this province and no amount of misrepresentation and maligning of these Crown Corporations by my opponent of the Liberal Party is going to divert the people of Saskatchewan from going on with the task of building the kind of Co-operative Commonwealth that my opponent started out to build but then lost heart and fell by the wayside.

Mr. Chairman: Ladies and gentlemen. I would like to thank and compliment this audience for their generally courteous attention to each speaker. I would like to congratulate both speakers for generally adhering to the subject under debate. It has made my duties as Chairman not only a privilege, but a pleasure.

30

Critical Analysis

Consensus was mixed as to the outcome of the debate. The media felt that Premier Douglas had certainly held his own. The media also felt that Thatcher had presented his case in a well-structured manner.

What the debate boiled down to was two politicians exchanging accounting numbers. They each offered their own numbers to support their respective political positions: Douglas in favor of Crown Corporations, Thatcher opposed.

It was surprising that Douglas did not take the opportunity to regale the audience with one of his colorful metaphors such as the Mouseland story or the Cream Separator economics story. Where was the humorous Douglas of past public speaking events? This debate would have been the perfect venue for a story to make the audience laugh and to put his opponent off guard.

Douglas was on slippery footing from the start of the debate, even acknowledging that he was hearing some booing from the crowd. Defensively, he wondered aloud if the booing was the sound of the sheep that former Premier Jimmy Gardiner had purchased for $100,000; a comment that angered the audience, prompting one observer to demand that Douglas get back on track talking about Crown Corporations.

Douglas then launched headlong into a focus on surplus and deficit numbers from the various Crown entities. While these numbers meant something to him, he perhaps should have given more thought to the average person in the audience who may not have grasped the significance of the various numbers being touted.

The first Crown that Douglas commented on was the Housing Corporation. The numbers he cited were accurate, however, what he failed to mention was that the numbers he cited were from 1947, some eight years prior. He explained that although the corporation showed a deficit of $42,400, there really was a surplus of $90,700. He explained that the surplus was due to monies received from the federal Canada Mortgage and Housing Corporation. Surpluses. Deficits. Eight-year-old data. Did Douglas really expect the audience to grasp what he was referring to?

Douglas then went on to mention how Thatcher, in his House of Commons remarks, failed to mention the Saskatchewan Reconstruction Corporation which had turned a profit. Perhaps Douglas should have cited specific examples of how this profitable entity had yielded impressive benefits to many Saskatchewan communities by repurposing wartime structures into local community halls and local curling rinks.

Douglas then focused on Thatcher's comments about the Fish Marketing Board. This quickly led to a series of observations about guaranteed floor prices for fish. Did the audience fully grasp the subject of floor prices? Judging from the numbers cited by Douglas, it appears that Thatcher's comments were valid. The government was using taxpayer money to provide northern fishermen with a guaranteed income, all while not recording these expenses against the Fish Marketing Board.

Douglas then went on to correct an erroneous statement made by Thatcher concerning the amount of money that had been advanced to the Estevan Brick Plant; he pointed out that by the end of fiscal 1956, the plant was operating in the black. Did the audience fully understand this rapid-fire release of accounting numbers? Perhaps he would have been better off leaving the numbers out of the argument.

Douglas then set the record straight in regards to sodium sulphate operations. He noted that there had been plants at Palo (west of Biggar), Gladmar (south of Radville), and Ormeaux (west of Prince Albert). Nowhere in the financial statements reviewed at the Legislative Library was there a reference to these locations. Douglas' remarks concerning the Bishopric location near Mossbank do, however, align with the data in the financial statements. Instead of rattling off locations where there had been plants, Douglas perhaps should have focused on explaining to the audience what sodium sulphate was and what it was used for in industry.

Douglas then set the record straight on the Saskatchewan Transportation Company but he did not explain why his government had decided to push Greyhound and other small entrepreneurs out of business to make way for the Crown entity.

Douglas then went on to defend the finances of the Saskatchewan Government Insurance Office (now SGI). His comments regarding insurance package policies were not explained fully and he complicated his argument unnecessarily by talking about breaking the prairie provinces into two zones. Again, Douglas failed to remember that the audience in the room did not have the intimate understanding of the numbers that he did. He should have told the audience how much money had been given out in fiscal 1956 to settle insurance claims; numbers that the audience would have understood.

Douglas appeared to find his footing late in his allotted 40 minutes, suggesting Mr. Thatcher had made negative comments in the House of Commons concerning the Saskatchewan Crowns as a ploy to show Prime Minister St. Laurent that indeed Ross Thatcher was a genuine Liberal convert. Douglas made the claim that Thatcher had deserted the CCF voters who had sent him to Ottawa to serve as their MP. *This* was Tommy Douglas the orator, the story teller. But was it too late?

Instead of continuing his line of attack on Thatcher's loyalty, Douglas then fumbled badly when he suddenly veered off course and suggested that Thatcher was in possession of confidential documents from the RCMP pertaining to people within the CCF Party. Douglas did not suggest who these Party members might have been. There was no room in a debate about Crown Corporations to entertain allegations of spying. The debate chairman was quick to realize this, and cautioned the Premier to get back on point. In any debate, leveling an unsubstantiated personal attack on your opponent is an indication of weakness. To audience members, it must have appeared as through Thatcher was getting under the skin of Douglas.

Thanks to declassification of federal documents in the early 1980s, the allegations that Douglas made are now better understood. It turns out that Douglas had been one of those spied on by the RCMP from the late 1930s through the 1980s. The RCMP's primary mission was to discover whether he had ties to the Communist Party of Canada. A 1980 internal assessment of the dossier states: *Douglas has been known personally by and has associated with leftists, peace movement workers and Communist Party of Canada members for years. He has allowed his name to stand publicly on many occasions in relation to support of issues sponsored by leftist groups.* Material in the RCMP file goes on to say: *It is difficult to determine the full depth of sympathy and involvement or influence, if any, these groups or their philosophies have over him.* The assessment concluded that, *there is much we do not know about Douglas and the file should be maintained in order to correlate any additional information that surfaces which might assist in piecing this jigsaw puzzle together.*

In any confrontational argument, or debate, it helps to bring calm to the event by offering empathy to your opponent. Thatcher could have started the debate by blasting the Premier for alleging inappropriate behavior with regards to files form the RCMP Instead, in his opening comments, Mr. Thatcher showed empathy when he said, "I felt a moment ago that perhaps the Premier was a little bitter. I can't say that I blame him for not talking about Crown Corporations at all in the last 10 minutes of his speech because the record is pretty bad."

Thatcher could then have gone on to tear apart the Crown Corporations. Instead, he offered more empathy admitting in the beginning he had been an enthusiastic believer in the Crown program. Perfect. The crowd was now listening intently to Thatcher.

Thatcher's debate performance was well polished. He came to the event prepared and delivered his argument in a reasoned manner. Instead of launching into a litany of surplus and deficit figures, Thatcher demonstrated that he was aware that the audience had just been treated to a recitation of accounting numbers from Douglas.

Thatcher told the audience that he was going to explore three questions pertaining to the Crowns: Were the Crowns efficient? Have the Crowns provided jobs? Have they provided revenue to the Treasury for social service type projects? He said these questions would reveal whether state socialism in Saskatchewan had succeeded or failed.

In any debate or speech to a group of assembled people, it helps to describe the key factors that will be discussed. This motivates the audience to pay attention. By taking this approach, and delineating three key questions, Thatcher quickly gained the audience's undivided attention.

To begin, Thatcher summarized the outcome of the tannery, shoe factory, and wool factory operations. The numbers cited were all accurate and supported his premise that socialism had failed.

He then took a swing at the Housing Corporation. But he slipped when he focused on an accounting nuance, which people likely did not grasp. He then compared the housing units that had been created to a slum. This was a personal opinion that he could not quantify. Perhaps he should have avoided any reference to the Housing Corporation if he could not make a more powerful argument.

He next targeted the Fish Board. He referred to some of the accounting numbers for the fishing venture as "little more than fiction." The numbers he cited are all correct and support his premise that socialism had failed. His attack on the Prince Albert box factory was also supported with accurate numbers.

The Estevan Brick Plant presented Thatcher with a hurdle. While the plant had some start-up difficulties, it had managed to erase its initial deficits. Thatcher's only angle of attack was that the brick plant had not made any interest payments on the initial advances from the Finance department. This was a weak argument to support a premise that socialism had failed. Thatcher would have been better off to avoid any discussion of the brick plant.

His argument of socialism being a failure further faltered when he admitted that the Government Printing Company was making money. He then further conceded that Saskatchewan Telephone Company was also making money.

He next addressed the Timber Board. His argument was that it had forced private sawmills out of business. He failed to quantify this statement with actual data. He was likely very aware that after 1952, the timber venture had made money, hence his lack of supporting data. Where he missed an opportunity for a more pointed attack was when he chose not to address the sawmill at Big River which had been plagued with operational difficulties.

Thatcher next focused criticism on the Fur Marketing Service. He described how in the 1955-56 season, the government allowed trappers the option of selling their furs to whomever they wanted. He made this sound like the Fur Marketing Service had failed. In fact, it was changing consumer fashion trends that were negatively impacting fur prices that prompted the government to alter their approach. What he stopped short of admitting is that the Fur Marketing Service had brought economic activity to the north and had streamlined the business of fur in Saskatchewan.

Thatcher next addressed the Saskatchewan Government Insurance Office. He claimed that there was $9.6 million of liabilities on the Balance Sheet. Reviews of financial statements at the Legislative Library have been unable to identify any such liability figure. Thatcher then admitted that some of his other criticisms of the Insurance Office were incorrect. To save face, he then stated that in 1956 the Crown had lost $132,000. What he failed to explain was that in 1956 it was the general insurance part of the business that had lost money. Fire insurance premiums for that year had been reduced which prompted more customers to take out fire insurance policies. Unfortunately, there was an increase in fire insurance claims in 1956 which resulted in an underwriting loss. This in no way is related to government ownership. Thatcher was trying to throw a negative figure at the audience in hopes that they would grasp onto it.

Thatcher next addressed the Saskatchewan Transportation Company. This is where he regained his footing. In a bold move, he announced that there was in the audience one of the local entrepreneurs who had been displaced when the Crown entity was created. Weak profit numbers were then cited. What Thatcher carefully avoided was the fact that the Saskatchewan Transportation Company had been remitting small amounts of surplus funds back to the Finance department.

Thatcher then pursued a harsh line of attack against power and natural gas. He cited the three-year-old example of 50 farmers in the Crestwynd area (south of Moose Jaw) who were getting power from National Light and Power because Saskatchewan Power was too busy to bring service to them. National Light and Power had expressed a willingness to provide these farmers with power at a rate cheaper than what Saskatchewan Power could offer. The government granted National the permission to bring power to the area but on the condition that National charge a rate equal to that of Saskatchewan Power. Thatcher perhaps should have focused more intently on this Crestwynd situation. It is curious that none of these farmers seem to have been present at the debate. Or, if they were, Thatcher did not acknowledge their presence.

Thatcher made it a point to tell the audience that power rates in Saskatchewan were around 70% higher than in Manitoba. He was trying to shock the audience and build his argument that the Crowns were *not* efficient. He failed to reveal that power generation in Manitoba is created by hydroelectric dams on the Red River, a different economic situation than in Saskatchewan where electricity is mainly generated by coal-fired generating plants. All in all, not a fair comparison. Douglas seized on this unfair comparison in his rebuttal.

In a further bid to create an argument of inefficiency, Thatcher employed a similar numbers comparison strategy when he cited natural gas price differentials between Moose Jaw, Calgary, Medicine Hat, and Edmonton. Once again, Douglas called him on it during rebuttal by reminding the audience that Alberta had installed natural gas distribution pipelines several decades earlier. The infrastructure was now paid for and rates to customers were priced to reflect this. Thatcher should have known the dangers of placing misleading emphasis on numbers. He should have known that it was dangerous to expose one's flank to the likes of a seasoned politician like Douglas.

Thatcher then described how the Crown entities were not paying interest on monies advanced from the Finance department. They were also not paying for audit expenses, nor were they contributing to the cost of operating the Finance department. All these allegations were true. The

Crowns were not entirely paying their way entirely. Thatcher itemized the interest, auditing, and general expenses that had been shouldered by general taxpayer revenues. During the debate, Douglas carefully avoided setting foot in this issue. Perhaps Thatcher should have focused more intently on the use of taxpayer funds to pay some of the Crown operating expenses. Perhaps Thatcher should have labeled his criticism as one of "two sets of books."

To explore his question of whether or not the Crowns had created jobs, Thatcher offered Bureau of Statistics data that showed a distinct lack of manufacturing sector jobs had been created in the province. Douglas called him on this statement and reminded the audience that the Bureau only gathered data on manufacturing firms greater than a certain size. Douglas then pointed out that if all economic sectors were considered, the province had created more than 10,000 jobs since 1944.

To build on his final question of whether the Crowns had provided any money for social services, roads, or education, Thatcher suggested that no money from any Crown Corporation had found its way into such programs. While he offered no supporting evidence for this statement, reviews of financial statements in the Legislative Library show that on occasion money generated from Timber Board operations was used to pay for road creation in northern areas. One would have to dig very deep into budgetary cash flows to determine where funds remitted from the other Crowns to the Finance department ultimately ended up. It seems that Thatcher was, on balance, correct in his assertion.

There is one mathematical opportunity that Thatcher failed to thoroughly seize upon. At one point, Douglas stated that to the end of 1955, the province had invested $9,634,000 in the various Crown Corporations. In fiscal 1955, the Crowns recorded a collective surplus of $1,366,000. Douglas reasoned this was a 14.18% return on investment. He made it sound as if this 14.18% was for 1955 alone. It was not. The surplus was for the ten-year period 1945 to 1955. This equates to something closer to 1.4% per year. Perhaps Thatcher legitimately missed this opportunity. Perhaps he recognized the opportunity, but was gracious enough to save Douglas the embarrassment. In either case, the mathematical returns of the overall Crown Corporation strategy left much to be desired. Had Thatcher hammered on this bit of math, he might have walked away the decisive winner.

In his 10-minute rebuttal, Douglas had one brilliant moment that underscored his oratory skills. He said in a zinger of a comment "I say to my Liberal friends here, we (the CCF) had him yesterday, you've got him today, heaven only knows who will have him tomorrow." This was a suggestion that Ross Thatcher would not be loyal for long to the Liberal Party.

This was a difficult debate as any debate involving a recitation of accounting numbers is likely to be. The numbers presented were presented in a rapid-fire manner. The audience members, including the media, were not intimately versed in Crown Corporation accounting. Mr. Thatcher on a few occasions left his hind flank exposed to stinging rebuttal from Douglas. Premier Douglas made a tactical error when he veered off into an attack against Thatcher regarding RCMP files.

But in the end, it was not Premier Douglas who was seeking election. It was Ross Thatcher. So, was there a winner? Was there a loser?

After the audience had disbursed, Gravelbourg MLA, Leo Coderre commented to the media, "This is exactly what the Party needed. Someone had to show that Douglas is mortal, that he is just another politician, and that he is not invincible. Thatcher did that tonight and it could be a turning point for us."

A Calgary Herald journalist who attended the event later wrote, *Ross Thatcher emerged from the debate as a new power in Saskatchewan politics, not because he won, but because he didn't lose.*

But in the end, it would be the people of the Assiniboia riding that would serve as judge and jury. CCF incumbent Hazen Argue picked up 10,389 votes. Liberal candidate Ross Thatcher picked up 8,862 votes. And with that, Mr. Thatcher's time in Ottawa was done. His gamble of switching to the Liberal Party had failed.

- This was a difficult debate. The subject matter revolved around numbers that the audience members would not have been familiar with.
- There was no decisive winner of the debate. Both men made tactical errors in their deliveries. This debate highlighted that all men are fallible, even politicians.
- The debate did however change the way politics is done in Canada. This debate brought politics to the people. For those who could not attend in person, radio broadcasts brought the event into people's homes. The next time you witness an all-party debate on television, think back to Mossbank in 1957.
- There are many questions that will go unanswered in the history books concerning this debate including: Should it have occurred in the first place? Instead of debating Premier Douglas, would Mr. Thatcher have been further ahead in challenging his CCF opponent, Hazen Argue, to a debate?

31

Ross Thatcher
Comes Home

In Ottawa, the 1957 election was a shake-up for the Liberal Party as a whole. John Diefenbaker, the rising political star from Prince Albert, Saskatchewan, saw his Conservative Party take 112 seats. The St. Laurent Liberals could only muster 105 seats. The CCF Party held its own, taking 25 seats (a gain of two from the last election). Ten of these seats were in Saskatchewan, where it seemed the people were not ready to turn away the CCF. Was Mr. Thatcher too hasty in breaking ranks with the CCF? Had he run in his Moose Jaw riding on the CCF ticket he may well have been returned to Ottawa. In fact, the Moose Jaw riding saw former Moose Jaw mayor L.H. Lewry score a decisive win on the CCF ticket.

Thatcher was quick to realize that Diefenbaker had only a minority government and that there would be another federal election soon. In the 1958 election, Thatcher decided to stand on the Liberal ticket once again in the Assiniboia riding. This time, however, the results were even worse. CCF incumbent Hazen Argue powered to victory with 9,104 votes. The Conservative candidate, W.J. Ferguson scored 6,360 votes, and Thatcher garnered 6,173 votes. The stage lights were dimming. The curtain was closing on Ross Thatcher's federal political ambitions.

1960

It was time for Ross Thatcher to plot his next moves. He set his sights on the Saskatchewan provincial Liberal scene where Alexander Hamilton "Hammy" McDonald was leader. In 1948, Hammy was elected to the Saskatchewan Legislature in the Moosomin riding. He held this riding for five consecutive elections. But his leadership was coming under scrutiny. The Liberal Party was struggling financially and had little money in the bank. Its energy had been zapped by successive Douglas CCF wins. Questions were being asked about McDonald's inability to raise money for Party coffers.

Thatcher's performance in the Mossbank debate had many in the provincial Liberal organization paying attention. What if Thatcher could bring his skills and abilities to help the provincial Liberals? Could the Liberals oust the CCF government under a Thatcher-led Liberal Party? Thatcher turned his attention to fund-raising for the provincial Liberals. His hardware store was making money as was his cattle operation. He had just purchased a hardware store in Saskatoon and another in Regina. Ross Thatcher had little to worry about, except getting back into politics.

Hammy McDonald could feel the pressures mounting; criticism began to swirl that he lacked energy and drive. In the summer of 1959, he was firmly at odds and on the defensive with the provincial Liberal Party. He cited health reasons and stepped away from the Party leadership.

McDonald's exit necessitated a leadership convention, and Ross Thatcher won the leadership role on the first ballot. He was back on the political stage. Soon enough, so too would Hammy McDonald. In May 1965, McDonald headed to Ottawa, this time to take up a Senate seat.

HEALTHCARE

In a drive to implement a healthcare mechanism, Douglas called an election for June of 1960. It was time for Ross Thatcher in his new role as Liberal Party leader to step up and shine. In the 1960 provincial election, Thatcher ran in the riding of Morse (west of Moose Jaw). It was a close contest. Thatcher took 2,791 votes, with his CCF competitor nipping at his heels with 2,629 votes.

The CCF won the election, taking 38 seats. But the Liberals scored 16 seats and realized an uptick in the popular vote. Despite having been just elected, Thatcher's focus was already solidly on the next provincial election. He immediately got to work on a polarization effort. The way he saw it, the Saskatchewan electorate had to be given a stark choice: left wing socialism or right-wing free enterprise. He would tell the electorate that he had looked socialism up close in the eye and decided it was not viable. So much so that he had left the CCF Party. He figured that when presented with this clear left-right choice, a Saskatchewan Liberal government would be the result.

Thatcher began recruiting new Party members. He wooed Social Credit members. He made efforts to strengthen his relation with Conservative members, particularly the Conservative leader Martin Pederson. Soon enough, Thatcher would be able to test his efforts in real time.

In February 1961, a by-election was called in the riding of Turtleford. The 1960 election in the Turtleford riding had seen CCF candidate Bob Wooff beat incumbent Liberal Frank Foley by 12 votes. A court challenge resulted in the election being nullified and a by-election being called. The results of the by-election were clear. Liberal Frank Foley won by a 600-vote margin. Ross Thatcher was elated. His message was starting to resonate.

Meanwhile, momentum was building towards the Douglas government implementing a Medicare policy. In November 1961, the legislation was finally passed. Medicare would take effect in July of 1962. Saskatchewan now would have government-controlled, universal medical insurance – the first of its kind in North America.

With the passing of this legislation, Douglas had realized a political pinnacle. He then made the monumental decision to step away from provincial politics. He had just been named the new leader of the federal NDP Party. He was off to Ottawa again. The CCF Party appointed Woodrow Lloyd as Party leader. By default, Lloyd also became the new Premier of Saskatchewan.

With Douglas on his way to Ottawa, a by-election was called for December 1961 to fill his vacancy in the Weyburn riding. Liberal Herbert Staveley beat CCF candidate Oran Reiman by just over 800 votes. The hallowed, revered Weyburn riding had fallen to a Liberal. Thatcher could feel the ground shifting.

Thatcher was not necessarily opposed to the idea of Medicare. While he shunned the CCF Party, he had not lost his social conscience. He aimed his attacks at the CCF Medicare plan, stressing that Premier Woodrow Lloyd was being arrogant in his discussions with doctor associations who were opposed to Medicare. He took particular aim at the Medical Care Insurance Commission the Lloyd government had established as the sole agency for dealing with doctors. Thatcher referred to the Commission as "vicious compulsion" and "peacetime conscription of the medical profession." He reminded people that they were now seeing "economic strangulation." He warned that if the CCF government could take away Doctors rights, then other organizations were also at risk.

Another political test came in 1962 when the CCF MLA from the Prince Albert riding, Lachlan Fraser McIntosh, died. In the ensuing by-election, Liberal candidate David Steuart trounced the CCF candidate by 2,400 votes. That was three for three. The momentum had shifted in the Liberals' favour.

PREMIER ROSS THATCHER

In the April 1964 election, Thatcher was once again successful in his Morse riding, but only by a margin of 236 votes. Province-wide, however, the Liberals' message prevailed and with that, Ross Thatcher was the Premier of Saskatchewan. Thatcher won in his Morse riding again in the 1967 election when his Liberals again prevailed province-wide.

During his tenure as Premier, he courted big industry and attracted capital for potash development, and pulp and paper mill mills in the north. But he also governed on a platform of capital spending reduction and waste elimination. He reduced taxes and sold off some minor Crown Corporations. He was, however, careful to retain the larger Crowns for fear of alienating voters. In other words, the politician who in 1956-1957 hammered the efficiency of the Crown Corporations was just that – a politician. He knew the voters would not warm to any plan to eliminate the Crowns. He knew any such platform would be dangerous to his re-election chances.

Thatcher made his opposition to unionized labour abundantly clear. In 1966, when 1,200 unionized workers at Saskatchewan Power went on strike demanding an 8% wage increase, Thatcher called an emergency session of the legislature. The striking workers were labeled as an essential service and ordered back to work. The provincial *Trade Union Act* was subsequently amended such that strikes had to be approved by a majority of union members, not a majority of those who voted. Thatcher was hoping his actions would resonate with private enterprise mulling whether or not to invest in Saskatchewan.

On a softer note, Thatcher devoted attention to the Indigenous population in the province. He ordered the Public Service to have at least 5% its people of Indigenous background and to provide them with necessary job training. Dental issues also were important with Thatcher. He ordered the Health Department to take action; the result was the creation of the College of Dentistry in Saskatoon.

In 1967, Thatcher sought another mandate from the people. The unemployment rate had fallen and jobs were being created. Oil production was up. Potash production was growing at a 25% clip, uranium mining was a going concern, and capital investment across the entire resource sector was rising. Saskatchewan was poised to become a "have" province. But Saskatchewan was still largely an agrarian province and on world markets the price of wheat was softening. In the early 1960s, wheat was trading at over $2 per bushel but in 1967 price was in a downtrend, headed for $1.25 per bushel. Farmers were not happy. Nevertheless, on balance, the people decided Thatcher was doing a good job. The Liberals gained three seats over the last election to now hold 35.

But something was wrong. Thatcher's outlook had suddenly changed. Mere days after the election, Thatcher convened his Cabinet and abruptly announced that he had heard from Ottawa that a recession was imminent. To avoid getting caught in its crosshairs, he decided to implement across-the-board austerity plans. Thatcher also feared that socialist tentacles might take root in the province. In the US, the late 1960s were a time of anti-Vietnam War protests and anti-establishment rhetoric. To prevent this thinking from infiltrating into Saskatchewan, Thatcher took the unusual step of ordering immediate cuts to education funding. To reduce government outlays on healthcare, he implemented what he termed "deterrence fees" on medical visits. It would now cost $1.50 to see a doctor and $2.50 a day to stay in the hospital. Thatcher's Ministers were not happy. He became increasingly combative with them and would not budge off his austerity plans.

Ottawa's prognosis for a recession proved true. Grain prices fell, potash prices fell, and inflation became a serious concern. In fact, the potash industry was in a mess thanks to its overproduction. Thatcher created the Potash Conservation Board. All potash producers would be expected to adhere to government dictated production levels. This from the same Ross Thatcher who had railed against government involvement in industry during the 1957 Mossbank debate.

In Ottawa, Pierre Trudeau's Liberal government decided the best way to counter falling wheat prices was to grow less. Wheat Board Minister, Saskatchewan MP Otto Lang, implemented the L.I.F.T. Program. The details were complex, but boiled down to farmers making a decision to grow wheat and sell it into a soft market or accept a per-acre incentive payment to not grow grain. Neither option held appeal for Saskatchewan farmers. They expressed their distaste for Liberals, both provincially and federally.

Thatcher called an election in June 1971 seeking a fresh mandate from the people. But former CCF bureaucrat Alan Blakeney and his NDP Party were ready. The NDP soundly defeated the Liberals, reducing their seats to 15. Thatcher won his Morse riding again, but the lights were dimming on his provincial political career. The public had rejected his leadership and he announced he would be stepping down as Party leader.

Three weeks later, on July 22 1971, Ross Thatcher unexpectedly died of a heart at his home in Regina.

- Ross Thatcher decided to try once again to win election in the riding of Assiniboia in the 1960 federal election. But again, the constituents denied him victory.
- Thatcher turned his attention to fund raising for the provincial Liberals. His performance in Mossbank had many wondering if he was the answer to forming a Liberal government in Saskatchewan.
- In the 1960 provincial election, Thatcher eked out a narrow

victory in the riding of Morse. He immediately got to work telling the people of Saskatchewan they had a choice: left-wing socialism or right-wing free enterprise.

- In the 1964 provincial election, Thatcher again won his Morse seat by a slim margin. The Liberals prevailed as well across the province. Ross Thatcher was now Premier Thatcher.
- He turned his attention to capital spending reduction and waste elimination, selling some Crown Corporations and reducing taxes. He courted big industry and attracted capital for potash development, and pulp and paper mill construction in the north. In 1967, the Liberals were again returned to office.
- Following the 1967 election, Thatcher shifted his focus to a platform of austerity, fearing that a recession was on the horizon.
- Ross Thatcher called an election in June 1971 seeking a fresh mandate. But former CCF bureaucrat Alan Blakeney and the NDP party soundly defeated the Liberals, reducing their seats to 15. Thatcher won his Morse riding, but the lights were dimming on his provincial political career. The stress was taking its toll.
- Three weeks later, on July 22 1971, Ross Thatcher unexpectedly died of a heart at his home in Regina.

32

Tommy Douglas
Returns to Ottawa

The electoral shift away from the St. Laurent Liberals in 1957 helped the CCF Party gain two seats in the House of Commons to now hold a total of 25. But the support was to be short-lived.

In 1958, the Diefenbaker Conservatives powered to a landslide victory, taking 208 seats. The Liberals under new leader Lester Pearson only managed to win 48 seats. The CCF Party was humiliated, taking only eight seats. Only one of these seats was from Saskatchewan; Hazen Argue in the Assiniboia riding. The CCF Party, in a bid to remain viable at the federal level, decided to expand its base to by appealing to organized labour. The Canadian Labour Congress was approached about forming a new national party.

Meanwhile, in Saskatchewan, the Douglas government tabled and passed the *Medical Care Insurance Act*. Douglas felt he had the wind at his back with the Diefenbaker federal government indicating it was generally in favour of what Saskatchewan was doing on the healthcare front. This sentiment came because John Diefenbaker's mother was permanently hospitalized in Prince Albert. Diefenbaker fully appreciated the benefits of an improved healthcare system, not only in Saskatchewan, but across Canada. However, the Diefenbaker government stopped short of providing the funding needed to institute a true national hospital insurance program. Instead, the Diefenbaker government established a Royal Commission on Health Services in 1961 to further study national medical care. The final report released in 1965 recommended Medicare for all of Canada.

Douglas reasoned that the first order of business within the new Act would be to have the government pay doctors for patient visitations. An Advisory Committee visited seven countries around the world and held both public and private hearings on doctor compensation. The Committee tabled its report on September 25, 1961. The report recommended that doctors be paid $1 for seeing a patient in their office and $2 for a home visit.

In 1961, the federal CCF Party re-imagined itself in the form of the New Democratic Party (NDP). Major Coldwell had been defeated in the 1958 federal election in his Rosetown-Biggar riding. Hazen Argue had been elected as Party leader. Several key players in the NDP were openly calling for Douglas to re-enter the federal arena. They argued that the NDP needed someone dynamic at the helm. They expressed concern that the Party had become divided into two camps: labour and farmer. They felt that Hazen Argue was too closely aligned to farmers. They felt they needed a leader who would appeal to farmer and unionized labourer alike. Major Coldwell reminded Tommy Douglas that he was a natural fit for the leadership. He was reminded of his prior experience in Ottawa politics, how he had made significant healthcare policy advances in Saskatchewan, and that he was an eloquent and effective speaker.

The decision to re-enter the political sphere in Ottawa was a difficult one. Douglas felt a draw to remain in Saskatchewan politics to thoroughly roll out the new *Medical Care Insurance Act*.

After much thought, he concluded that the shift to federal politics would be straightforward enough, aided by the recently-passed *Medical Care Insurance Act*. At the Party convention in August 1961, Douglas, received 1,391 votes and Hazen Argue 380 votes. In his victory speech he invoked some lines from English poet, William Blake, "I shall not cease from mental fight / Nor shall my sword sleep in my hand / Till we have built Jerusalem / In this green and pleasant land."

Douglas decided he would run in the riding of Regina-City on the NDP ticket in what was expected to be a 1962 federal election.

But the political winds had shifted in a dangerous direction. Shortly after Saskatchewan introduced the *Medical Care Insurance Act,* Britain created its own program called the National Health Service (NHS). Doctors in the UK cried foul and began exiting the country heading for places like Canada. They would not practice socialized medicine.

As many of these UK doctors landed in Canada, the opposition to a socialized medicine scheme intensified. The province's doctors, began insisting on a multi-payer approach. They wanted people to have private insurance. If the government wanted to subsidize those who absolutely could not afford insurance, then so be it, but the doctors envisioned a system where the majority of people would have private insurance. Opposition to the government plan went far beyond just a few doctors. The College of Physicians and Surgeons of Saskatchewan mounted an expensive publicity campaign that was supported by both the Canadian Medical Association and the American Medical Association. The campaign roused the general public by asking whether people wanted "Dictators or Doctors." The campaign language even resorted to words like *totalitarianism*.

In the June 1962 federal election, the NDP more than doubled their 1958 seat count, taking 19. But, there was a problem. Douglas's political gatherings in the Regina-City riding had been poorly attended. The doctors announced they intended to go on strike. The electorate was riled up over the potential for a doctor's strike. The voters took out their frustrations the best way they knew how; using the ballot box. NDP Party leader, Tommy Douglas failed to win election in the Regina riding. Regina businessman Ken More scored 22,164 votes. Tommy Douglas could only muster 12,736 votes. At his concession speech, Tommy Douglas cited the words of a Scottish ballad, "Fight on my men. I am hurt, but not slain. I'll lie me down to bleed awhile, but then I will rise and fight again."

And fight again, he did. Erhart Regier, the NDP MP for the B.C. riding of Burnaby-Coquitlam, resigned so that Tommy Douglas could run in a by-election. Douglas won handily, scoring 22,553 votes to the Liberal candidate's 12,090 votes. With the by-election detour behind him, he was finally off to Ottawa.

But the once gleaming image of Tommy Douglas was now showing signs of tarnish. Behind closed doors in Ottawa, NDP MPs began to question their leader. Did he have the image to carry the Party forward? Could he improve his French language skills? He was a powerful orator on the radio, but could he muster that same appeal on the new technological medium of television?

In the federal election of April 1963, the Liberals won a minority government and the NDP lost several seats. In the 1965 federal election, the NDP clawed back some of what it had lost, taking 21 seats. In the House of Commons, Douglas kept pushing for national medical care. Finally in 1966, The Pearson government passed the *Medical Care Act* which provided for cost sharing between Ottawa and the provinces, not unlike what Saskatchewan had established several years earlier.

In the June 1968 federal election, a new phenomenon swept the land– Trudeaumania. The NDP took 22 seats, but Douglas lost in his newly redrawn riding of Burnaby-Seymour in a close contest. Douglas took 17,753 votes, but his Liberal competitor, Ray Perreault, narrowly squeezed past him with 17,891 votes.

Again, the by-election strategy came into play, this time under less pleasant circumstances. Colin Cameron, NDP MLA for the B.C. riding of Nanaimo-Cowichan-Islands, died suddenly of a stroke in July 1968. Douglas ran in the February 1969 by-election and won. Douglas took 19,730 votes and his Liberal rival, Eric Winch, 12,8907 votes. Having now relied on two by-elections to retain a seat in the Commons, it was apparent that it was time for a new NDP leader. It was agreed Douglas would stay at the helm until 1971.

Despite the electoral challenges, Tommy Douglas continued his crusade to make life better for all Canadians. His pressure on Prime Minister Trudeau helped bring about the Canada Pension Plan. With assistance behind the scenes from senior bureaucrat Albert Johnson (who at one time had worked for Douglas in Saskatchewan), Douglas pushed the Trudeau government towards a redesign of social security, and more federal funding for post-secondary education. Douglas also railed against Trudeau over the *War Measures Act*. In October 1970, the Front de Libération du Québec (FLQ) kidnapped British diplomat, James Richard Cross, along with Quebec's Minister of Labour, Pierre Laporte. After the Trudeau government invoked the *War Measures Act* which suspended civil liberties, the FLQ murdered Laporte. While Douglas condemned the killing, he described Trudeau's action as, "The government is using a sledgehammer to crack a peanut."

At the NDP convention held in Ottawa in April 1971, Douglas was succeeded by David Lewis. Tommy Douglas remained in Ottawa as MP for the riding of Nanaimo-Cowichan-Islands until 1979. At the age of 74, he decided it was time to retire.

In 1981, Douglas discovered that he had incurable cancer and on February 24, 1986 he died of cancer at his home in Ottawa. A giant in Canadian politics, the likes of which we may never see again, was gone.

In his political career that spanned 1935 through 1979, Tommy Douglas played a leadership role in:

- kickstarting the Saskatchewan economy in the post-war, post-depression years
- fighting the federal government for assistance to Saskatchewan farmers
- pushing the progress of the Saskatchewan Power Corporation to electrify rural Saskatchewan
- pushing the progress of Saskatchewan telephones to bring phone service to the rural areas
- passing legislation to protect farm families
- reforming labour laws in Saskatchewan
- introducing a Bill of Rights in Saskatchewan
- introducing the *Hospitalization Act*
- introducing the *Medical Care Act* of 1966
- advancing the principle that we are all in the world together and should look after each other and also look after the less fortunate.

Conclusion

Tommy Douglas realized the economic system had failed. In order to really help people, he stepped away from the pulpit, rolled up his sleeves and dove headlong into the world of politics.

Douglas was a resilient man. Perhaps this was related to his experiences as a boxer when he was younger. A failed attempt at securing a seat in the Saskatchewan legislature did not discourage him. He picked himself up, dusted himself off, and pursued a seat in Ottawa under the CCF Party.

As an MP in Ottawa, he argued tirelessly for federal help to struggling Saskatchewan farmers. He eventually found himself at odds with Party bosses over the darkening situation in Europe. He could not bear the pacifist ideals of the CCF Party. It was time to move on.

Douglas returned to Saskatchewan where he was soon named provincial CCF Party leader. In 1944, he ran in the Weyburn riding on the CCF ticket. His oratory skills, his drive, and his genuine concern for his fellow man created momentum sufficient to push the ruling Liberals out of the way.

As the Premier of Saskatchewan, he hired a team of educated, skilled bureaucrats and wasted little time in implementing new economic strategies. It may never be known for sure, but it is likely that the Douglas government was expecting a repeat of what had happened after World War I. Private enterprise was at a standstill as the world watched Germany struggle under the weight of forced monetary reparations. With private enterprise operating from a position of uncertainty, the economy suffered from shortages of all manner of consumer goods.

To avoid a repeat of the World War I situation, the Douglas bureaucrats acted quickly to set up a network of Crown Corporations. These companies would manufacture leather, shoes, and wool products. Fish and furs from the north part of Saskatchewan would be sold into the global market. The vast stands of timber in the north would be harvested and sawn into lumber and other forest products. Sodium sulphate would be extracted and sold to the textile industry and the pulp and paper industry. Wartime assets would be purchased cheaply from the federal government and resold at a profit to towns and villages across the province. Housing would be created for returning veterans. An airline service would be started, a bus company would be launched, a brick plant would be resurrected, a printing company would be launched, and an insurance company created.

No two economic dislocations are alike. The scenario of shortages that had been envisioned did not materialize. The *Bretton Woods Agreement* made America the de-facto global economic leader and the US dollar the global reserve currency. The *Marshall Plan* to rebuild Europe, and the Allied powers efforts to rebuild Japan caused American-led private enterprise to resume action, making products that they had skillfully been making prior to the war. The Douglas government had no way of knowing that this course of action would unfold.

In looking at the financial statements for many of these Crown entities, it becomes evident that trying to create manufacturing industries from a position of little or no experience in an economy where already-skilled private enterprises are operating was a dangerous mission. The Saskatchewan Crown Corporations engaged in manufacturing consumer goods soon found themselves up against a wall of difficulty and steep learning curves.

What the Douglas team perhaps should have done was to partner with private enterprise; not compete with it. But this would have placed the Douglas team offside with respect to CCF policy. It was a sticky situation. Walk away and hope that private enterprise would be able to find Saskatchewan on the map, or stay the course, abide by your ideals, and plough more money into the Crown entities that were ailing.

Aggression often breeds haste. Steering an economy through an economic dislocation is not an easy task. A desire to get things happening quickly is understandable. In their haste to create Crown Corporations, a box factory in Prince Albert was seized when the owner refused to cooperate with his unionized workforce. Greyhound Bus Lines and other smaller entrepreneurs were forced out of the way to make room for a transportation Crown Corporation. Fishermen were compelled to sell their catches through the Fish Marketing Board. Fur trappers and fur ranchers were compelled to do business through the Fur Service. Private enterprise was discouraged from getting involved in wood products. An airline service was created at significant cost. While some of these entities did make money, others did not. The social benefit of ploughing money into some of these ventures was questionable to start with. In other cases, the social benefit was immediately apparent, but soon faded.

On the service front, Saskatchewan Telephone Corporation and Saskatchewan Power Corporation had been created prior to the CCF government taking power. Telephone and electrification services were aggressively expanded across the province. The Douglas team made both general and auto insurance affordably available to Saskatchewan residents. These ventures were all successful.

However, on the whole, criticism must be tempered. Steering an economy through an economic dislocation is not an easy task. Present day governments are discovering this as they battle post-pandemic inflation brought on by monetary stimulus used to keep the economy afloat as COVID ravaged the globe. Governments had no way of peeking around the corner to see how long the pandemic would linger. They had to act, and they did so in the best way they knew how. Were their strategies all perfect? Certainly not.

Likewise, in 1944, the Douglas government could not peek around the corner and assess what lay ahead. The war would soon end; they knew that much. But the rest was uncertain. In the face of that uncertainty, and in alignment with Party ideals, they took action to give the Saskatchewan economy, with its agrarian focus, a swift boost. And action, they took. The question that will forever remain unanswered is—had the Liberals been elected again in 1944, what would they have done?

The uneven performance of the Saskatchewan Crowns caught the attention of Moose Jaw Liberal MP and hardware store magnate, Ross Thatcher. Much like Tommy Douglas a decade earlier, Thatcher was finding himself at odds with his CCF bosses in Ottawa. Sensing he had hit the end of the CCF road, he swung into action. He crossed the House of Commons floor from to join the Liberals. To impress his new political bosses, he spoke against the notion of public ownership of the planned Trans-Canada Pipeline by criticizing the Saskatchewan Crown Corporation program. He claimed public ownership was not viable and that the Saskatchewan Crowns were a dismal failure.

Premier Douglas fought back with harsh words of his own, calling Thatcher a liar and a traitor. The two men then agreed to a public debate in the Community Hall in the small farming town of Mossbank, located south of Moose Jaw. All would be welcome to come and witness; the media included. Both men delivered 40-minute speeches, each using his own interpretation of Crown Corporation financial performance to support their respective positions.

What both men shared was a deep concern for Saskatchewan. But their concerns were channeled along different ideological vectors. Tommy Douglas held a deep concern for the people. Ross Thatcher favored private enterprise, although he was not entirely at odds with the concept of Crown Corporations, provided they were run efficiently and created employment opportunities.

Douglas was not the one seeking election. He easily could have ignored Thatcher's harsh words in the House of Commons. Douglas did not have to debate anyone. He could have sat idly by while Thatcher battled CCF incumbent Hazen Argue in the Assiniboia riding. But such was his concern for Saskatchewan that Douglas could not allow someone to demean the Crown Corporations he and his team had started. Thatcher was clever and calculating. He knew if he issued derogatory words against Douglas' Crowns, he would incite some response. The idea of a debate was just what Thatcher was seeking. He needed a public performance to show people how much he cared for the province. He needed to show that he was committed to the Liberal ideals. May 20, 1957 in Mossbank would be Ross Thatcher's springboard into Liberal politics. Or, so he thought.

Both men fared reasonably well in the debate. But there was something different this time. Tommy Douglas was no longer the invincible politician. Ross Thatcher had managed, with little effort, to rattle Douglas. Douglas delivered a winded explanation of profits and losses in an effort to illustrate that his Crown entities had been successful. But he veered off unexpectedly and turned the debate personal, alleging that Thatcher had been working with the RCMP to gather information on people in the CCF Party. This was uncharacteristic of Douglas.

Unfortunately, for Ross Thatcher, the debate did not pan out as he expected. Although Thatcher presented a reasoned delivery of his view of Crown Corporations, it would not be enough. CCF incumbent Hazen Argue won re-election in the Assiniboia riding and Thatcher's days in Ottawa were over.

As for Douglas, the debate surely must have been a sign that he was no longer invincible. In an effort to keep up the fight, as any good boxer would do, he sharpened his focus and aimed his punches better. He decided to push full steam ahead on the Medicare file. He wanted better healthcare for the people of Saskatchewan. In 1960, he called an election seeking a fresh mandate. This would be his last provincial election. After putting in place the framework for Medicare, he left provincial politics and returned to Ottawa to lead the newly created NDP Party.

The debate humbled a sitting M.P. who had gambled on his future by switching sides in the House of Commons. Ross Thatcher returned to his hardware business, but kept a focus on politics. Realizing that he could be vulnerable on the political stage, he carefully regrouped himself and took another stab at politics, becoming the Premier of Saskatchewan in 1964. He served as Premier until his Party lost to the provincial NDP in 1971.

The 1957 Debate is often referred to as the "Great Debate". This was politics in action. This was politics brought to the people. The debate showcased a politician willing to stand up for his ideals when his own re-election was not even on the line. This debate showcased another politician who had switched political Parties out of care and concern for his province.

In a sense, the people of Saskatchewan were the winners of the 1957 Great Debate. The debate clearly showed that despite all his achievements, Douglas was not invincible; he was vulnerable to a poor showing. His performance motivated him to sharpen his focus and he aggressively began pursuit of a Medicare bill. Saskatchewan residents to this day remain the beneficiaries of his re-focused efforts.

I sincerely hope that that this book has enlightened you. I hope this book has whetted your appetite to learn more about both Saskatchewan and global geopolitics. I hope you now have a more illuminated view of not only Thatcher and Douglas, but also of the political atmosphere and events that led to the 1957 debate. I sincerely hope this book encourages you to read more about the political and economic events that have shaped the Province of Saskatchewan. I hope this book triggers your curiosity to learn more about the various politicians who played a role in making Saskatchewan what it is today— and perhaps to one day soon make a visit to the town of Mossbank, home of The Great Debate..

Notes

Chapter 1

Falkirk THI website. Available at: https://falkirkthi.com/our-falkirk-story.

Encyclopedia Britannica. Available at: https://www.britannica.com/topic/battle-of-Falkirk.

Encyclopedia Britannica. Available at: https://www.britannica.com/biography/Elizabeth-Stuart.

National Museums of Scotland. Available at:

https://www.nms.ac.uk/explore-our-collections/stories/scottish-history-and-archaeology/mary-queen-of-scots/mary-queen-of-scots/who-was-mary-queen-of-scots.

Anglotopia website. Available at: https://anglotopia.net/british-history/william-iii-william-mary-glorious-revolution.

Stewart, W. (2005) The Life and Political Times of Tommy Douglas, McArthur & Company, Toronto, Canada.

Shackleton, D. (1975) *Tommy Douglas, A Biography.* McLelland and Stewart, Toronto, Canada.

Chapter 2

Stewart, W. (2005) *The Life and Political Times of Tommy Douglas.* McArthur & Company, Toronto, Canada.

Shackleton, D. (1975) *Tommy Douglas, A Biography.* McLelland and Stewart, Toronto, Canada.

CBC Learning website (2001) *The Winnipeg General Strike.* Available at: https://www.cbc.ca/history/EPISCONTENTSE1EP12CH3PA2LE.html.

Jones, E. (2007) *Influenza 1918: Disease, Death, and Struggle in Winnipeg.* University of Toronto Press, Canada.

Johnson, E. (1979) *The Strikes in Winnipeg in May 1918.* The Prelude to 1919? M.A. Thesis, University of Manitoba.

West End Dumplings website (2013). Available at: http://westenddumplings.blogspot.com/2013/10/spanish-influenza-visits-manitoba.html.

Regehr, T.D. (2006). *Canadian Northern Railway.* Available at: https://www.thecanadianencyclopedia.ca/en/article/canadian-northern-railway.

Chapter 3

Stewart, W. (2005) *The Life and Political Times of Tommy Douglas.* McArthur & Company, Toronto, Canada.

Shackleton, D. (1975) *Tommy Douglas, A Biography.* McLelland and Stewart, Toronto, Canada.

Chapter 4

Stewart, W. (2005) *The Life and Political Times of Tommy Douglas.* McArthur & Company, Toronto, Canada.

Shackleton, D. (1975) *Tommy Douglas, A Biography.* McLelland and Stewart, Toronto, Canada.

Baird, C. (2021) *The History of Weyburn.* Canadian History Ehx website. Available at: https://canadaehx.com/2021/06/23/the-history-of-weyburn.

Encyclopedia of Saskatchewan. Available at: http://esask.uregina.ca/entry/palliser_and_hind_expeditions.html.

deBruin, T. (2019) *Tommy Douglas and Eugenics.* [Online]. Available at: https://www.thecanadianencyclopedia.ca/en/article/tommy-douglas-and-eugenics.

Leonard, T. (2016) *Illiberal Reformers; Race, Eugenics & American Economics in the Progressive Era.* Princeton University Press, USA.

Chapter 5

YouTube video (2014) *Greatest Canadian: Tommy Douglas.* Available at: https://youtu.be/g4_v2701GMg.

YouTube video (2006) *Prairie Giant: The Tommy Douglas Story.* Available at: https://youtu.be/bYyeYfzCRcs.

Watson, L. (2004) *She Was Never Afraid – The Biography of Annie Buller.* [Online] Available at: https://www.socialisthistory.ca/Docs/History/Buller/AB10.htm

Seager, A. (1977) *A History of the Mine Workers Union of Canada 1925-1936.* MA Thesis, March 1977, McGill University. Available at: https://escholarship.mcgill.ca/concern/theses/hx11xg294.

The Canadian Encyclopedia. [Online] Available at: https://www.thecanadianencyclopedia.ca/en/article/on-to-ottawa-trekregina-riot.

Canada History website. Available at: https://www.canadashistory.ca/explore/peace-conflict/the-regina-riot.

Chapter 6

Stewart, W. (2005) *The Life and Political Times of Tommy Douglas.* McArthur & Company, Toronto, Canada.

Shackleton, D. (1975) *Tommy Douglas, A Biography.* McLelland and Stewart, Toronto, Canada.

Smith, D. (2004) *James Gardiner. In: Saskatchewan Premiers of the 20th Century.* Ed. Gordon Barnhart. Canadian Plains Research Centre, Regina, SK.

Chapter 7

YouTube video (2006) *Prairie Giant: The Tommy Douglas Story.* Available at: https://youtu.be/bYyeYfzCRcs.

Canada History website (2021). *Woodsworth and the CCF.* Available at: https://www.canadahistory.com/sections/periods/Early_Canada/Depression/Woodsworth_and_the_CCF.html.

Chapter 8

Boyko, J. (2021) *The Regina Manifesto.* [Online] Available at: https://www.thecanadianencyclopedia.ca/en/article/regina-manifesto-1933.

Canadian Dimension website (2018) Full Text: *The CCFs Regina Manifesto.* https://canadiandimension.com/articles/view/the-regina-manifesto-1933-co-operative-commonwealth-federation-programme.

Chapter 9

Library of Parliament website. Available at: https://lop.parl.ca/sites/ParlInfo/default/en_CA/ElectionsRidings/Elections

Encyclopedia of Saskatchewan. Available at: https://esask.uregina.ca/entry/fines_clarence_melvin_1905-93.jsp

Chapter 10

YouTube video (2006) *Prairie Giant: The Tommy Douglas Story.* Available at: https://youtu.be/bYyeYfzCRcs.

Boyko, J. (2008) R.B. Bennett. [Online] Available at: https://www.thecanadianencyclopedia.ca/en/article/richard-bedford-viscount-bennett.

Stewart, W. (2005) *The Life and Political Times of Tommy Douglas.* McArthur & Company, Toronto, Canada.

Shackleton, D. (1975) *Tommy Douglas, A Biography.* McLelland and Stewart, Toronto, Canada.

Canada Info website. Available at: https://www.craigmarlatt.com/canada/government/king.html

Canada History Ehx website. Available at: https://canadaehx.com/2021/08/28/the-elections-1930.

Canada History Ehx website. Available at: https://canadaehx.com/2021/08/27/the-elections-1925-1926.

The Canadian Encyclopedia. Available at: https://www.thecanadianencyclopedia.ca/en/article/elections-of-1925-and-1926-feature.

Chapter 11

Neatby, H.B. (2008). *William Lyon McKenzie King.* The Canadian Encyclopedia. [Online] Available at: https://www.thecanadianencyclopedia.ca/en/article/william-lyon-mackenzie-king

Chapter 12

Encyclopedia of Saskatchewan. Available at: https://esask.uregina.ca/entry/williams george_1894-1945.jsp

Chapter 13

Encyclopedia of Saskatchewan. Available at: https://esask.uregina.ca/entry/patterson_william_john_1886-1976.jsp

Stewart, W. (2005) *The Life and Political Times of Tommy Douglas.* McArthur & Company, Toronto, Canada.

Shackleton, D. (1975) *Tommy Douglas, A Biography.* McLelland and Stewart, Toronto, Canada.

Smith, D. (2004) James Gardiner. In: *Saskatchewan Premiers of the 20th Century.* Ed. Gordon Barnhart. Canadian Plains Research Centre, Regina, SK

McLeod, T., McLeod, I. (2004) T.C. Douglas, In: *Saskatchewan Premiers of the 20th Century.* Ed. Gordon Barnhart. Canadian Plains Research Centre, Regina, SK.

Chapter 14

Eisler, D. (2004) Ross Thatcher. In: *Saskatchewan Premiers of the 20th Century.* Ed. Gordon Barnhart. Canadian Plains Research Centre, Regina, SK.

Eisler, D. (1987) *Rumours of Glory – Saskatchewan & the Thatcher Years.* Hurtig Publishers, Edmonton, Canada.

Chapter 17

Eisler, D. (2004) Ross Thatcher. In: *Saskatchewan Premiers of the 20th Century.* Ed. Gordon Barnhart. Canadian Plains Research Centre, Regina, SK.

Eisler, D. (1987) *Rumours of Glory – Saskatchewan & the Thatcher Years.* Hurtig Publishers, Edmonton, Canada.

Bodsworth, F. (1953). How Serious is the Defense Scandal? MacLean's Magazine. [Online] Available at: https://archive.macleans.ca/article/1953/2/1/how-serious-is-the-defense-scandal.

The Canadian Encyclopedia. [Online] Available at: https://www.thecanadianencyclopedia.ca/en/article/pipeline-debate

History.com website. Available at: https://www.history.com/topics/cold-war/suez-crisis

Encyclopedia of Saskatchewan. Available at: https://esask.uregina.ca/entry/argue_hazen_robert_1921-91.jsp

Chapter 19

Journals of the Legislative Assembly of the Province of Saskatchewan 1944-1956

Chapter 20

Journals of the Legislative Assembly of the Province of Saskatchewan 1944-1956

Chapter 21

Journals of the Legislative Assembly of the Province of Saskatchewan 1944-1956

Chapter 22

Journals of the Legislative Assembly of the Province of Saskatchewan 1944-1956

Chapter 23

Buhr, L. (1997) An Archeological Survey of Brick Manufacture in Saskatchewan. U of S. MA Thesis. Available at: https://www.collectionscanada.gc.ca/obj/thesescanada/vol2/SSU/TC-SSU-07302009105200.pdf

Sask Archives website. Available at: http://www.saskarchives.com/sites/default/files/documents/Elections-Results-by-Electoral-Division.pdf

Journals of the Legislative Assembly of the Province of Saskatchewan 1944-1956

Chapter 24

Journals of the Legislative Assembly of the Province of Saskatchewan 1944-1956

Chapter 25

Journals of the Legislative Assembly of the Province of Saskatchewan 1944-1956

Chapter 26

Journals of the Legislative Assembly of the Province of Saskatchewan 1944-1956

Chapter 28

Zado, P. (1980) *Furrows And Faith; A History Of Lake Johnston And Sutton R.M.'S. Expanse, Dunkirk, Bishopric, Mitchellton, Ardill, Mossbank, Vantage, Ettington, Mazenod, Palmer.* Published by Lake Johnston-Sutton Historical Society.

Chapter 29

Debate on Crown Corporations. Sourced from the Office of Carla Beck, MLA and Opposition Leader.

Chapter 31

Eisler, D. (2004) Ross Thatcher. In: *Saskatchewan Premiers of the 20th Century.* Ed. Gordon Barnhart. Canadian Plains Research Centre, Regina, SK.

Eisler, D. (1987) *Rumours of Glory – Saskatchewan & the Thatcher Years.* Hurtig Publishers, Edmonton, Canada.

Chapter 32

Briens, A.M. (2004) *The 1960 Saskatchewan Provincial Election.* M.A. degree thesis, University of Saskatchewan. Available at: https://ourspace. uregina.ca/handle/10294/13214.

McLeod, T., McLeod, I. (2004) T.C. Douglas, In: *Saskatchewan Premiers of the 20th Century.* Ed. Gordon Barnhart. Canadian Plains Research Centre, Regina, SK.

Stewart, W. (2005) *The Life and Political Times of Tommy Douglas.* McArthur & Company, Toronto, Canada.

Shackleton, D. (1975) *Tommy Douglas, A Biography.* McLelland and Stewart, Toronto, Canada.

Winchell, R.L. (1972) Farmer response to Lift, M.Sc. Thesis, University of British Columbia.[Online] Available at: https://open.library.ubc.ca/ soa/cIRcle/collections/ubctheses/831/items/1.0101553.

Waiser, B. (2006) *Tommy Douglas.* Fitzhenry & Whiteside, Markham. Canada.

About The Author

Malcolm Bucholtz holds on Engineering degree from Queen's University, and both an MBA and a M.Sc. degree from Heriot Watt University (Edinburgh, Scotland).

Malcolm is a researcher and author of more than twenty books on geopolitics, science, and the financial markets.

He lives in the small farming community of Mossbank, Saskatchewan.

www.ingramcontent.com/pod-product-compliance
Lightning Source LLC
Chambersburg PA
CBHW062123020426
42335CB00013B/1079